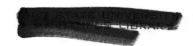

Genetic Technology and Sport

For elite athletes seeking a winning advantage, manipulation of their own genetic code has become a realistic possibility. In *Genetic Technology and Sport*, experts from sports science, genetics, philosophy, ethics and international sports administration describe the potential applications of the new technology and debate the questions surrounding its use:

- Genetic technology's implications for gender equality in sport
- Questions of definition: when am I a genetically enhanced athlete?
- The challenges facing international sports administration and testing laboratories

Genetic Technology and Sport is an accessible, informed and detailed exploration of the key issues surrounding sport and genetic modification. It raises profound moral and ethical questions about the value of sport, and vital practical questions about its governance. For sports professionals and administrators – and anyone concerned for the future of sport – this is essential reading.

Claudio Tamburrini is a Senior Researcher in the Department of Philosophy at Gothenburg University, Sweden. **Torbjörn Tännsjö** is Professor of Practical Philosophy at Stockholm University, Sweden.

Ethics and Sport

Series Editors
Mike McNamee
University of Wales, Swansea
Jim Parry
University of Leeds

The Ethics and Sport series aims to encourage critical reflection on the practice of sport, and to stimulate professional evaluation and development. Each volume explores new work relating to philosophical ethics and the social and cultural study of ethical issues. Each is different in scope, appeal, focus and treatment but a balance is sought between local and international focus, perennial and contemporary issues, level of audience, teaching and research application, and variety of practical concerns.

Also available in this series:

Ethics and Sport
*Edited by Mike McNamee and
Jim Parry*

Values in Sport
Elitism, nationalism, gender equality
and the scientific manufacture of
winners
*Edited by Torbjörn Tännsjö and
Claudio Tamburrini*

Spoilsports
Understanding and preventing
sexual exploitation in sport
Celia Brackenridge

Fair Play in Sport
A moral norm system
Sigmund Loland

Sport, Rules and Values
Philosophical investigations into
the nature of sport
Graham McFee

Sport, Professionalism and Pain
Ethnographies of injury and risk
David Howe

Genetically Modified Athletes
Biomedical ethics, gene doping
and sport
Andy Miah

Human Rights in Youth Sport
A critical review of children's
rights in competitive sports
Paulo David

Genetic Technology and Sport

Ethical questions

Edited by Claudio Tamburrini
and Torbjörn Tännsjö

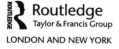

LONDON AND NEW YORK

First published 2005
by Routledge
2 Park Square, Milton Park, Abingdon, Oxon OX 14 4RN

Simultaneously published in the USA and Canada
by Routledge
270 Madison Ave, New York, NY 10016

Routledge is an imprint of the Taylor & Francis Group

Typeset in Goudy by
Keystroke, Jacaranda Lodge, Wolverhampton
Printed and bound in Great Britain by
MPG Books Ltd, Bodmin

British Library Cataloguing in Publication Data
A catalogue record for this book is available from the British Library

Library of Congress Cataloging in Publication Data
Tamburrini, Claudio Marcello.
  Genetic technology and sport : ethical questions / Claudio M Tamburrini and
Torbjörn Tännsjö
    p. cm. – (Ethics and sport)
  Includes bibliographical references and index.
  ISBN 0–415–34236–8 (hardback) – ISBN 0–415–34237–6 (pbk.) –
ISBN 0–203–48164–x (e book)
  1. Doping in sports. 2. Genetic engineering–Moral and ethical aspects. 3. Medical
genetics–Moral and ethical aspects. 4. Medial ethics. 5. Sports–Philosophy.
  I. Tännsjö, Torbjörn, 1946– II. Title. III. Series.
    RC1230.T362005
    362.29–dc22   2005005602

ISBN10: 0–415–34236–8   ISBN13: 9–78–0–415–34236–0 (Hbk)
ISBN10: 0–415–34237–6   ISBN13: 9–78–0–415–34237–7 (Pbk)

Contents

Notes on contributors

Lincoln Allison is Emeritus Reader in Politics at the University of Warwick and Visiting Professor in the Politics of Sport at the University of Brighton. From 1993 to 2002 he was Director of the Warwick Centre for the Study of Sport in Society. He has edited a number of books on the politics of sport and is the author of *Amateurism in Sport*. His other published academic work is mainly in the fields of environmental politics and political theory. He has also written and broadcast as a journalist, mainly in the fields of politics, sport and travel.

Gunnar Breivik is Professor of Social Sciences at Norwegian University of Sport and Physical Education (NUSPE). Since 1999 he has been Rector of NUSPE. His main research areas are in sport philosophy (phenomenology, ethics), sociology of sport (subcultures, value systems, activity patterns) and the psychology of sport (risk taking, extreme sports). He has published internationally in all areas.

Ruth Chadwick is Professor of Bioethics at Lancaster University, and Director of CESAGen, the ESRC Centre for Economic and Social Aspects of Genomics (a Lancaster–Cardiff collaboration). She co-edits the journal *Bioethics* and was editor-in-chief of the *Encyclopedia of Applied Ethics* (San Diego: Academic Press, 1998). Her most recent publication is R. Chadwick *et al.*, *Functional Foods* (Berlin: Springer-Verlag, 2003).

Simona Giordano is a Lecturer in Bioethics at the University of Manchester. She is the author of *Understanding Eating Disorders: Conceptual and Ethical Issues in the Treatment of Anorexia and Bulimia Nervosa* (Oxford University Press, in press). She has published on moral philosophy, the philosophy of psychiatry and bioethics.

John Harris is the Sir David Alliance Professor of Bioethics at the University of Manchester. His recent books include, as an editor, *Bioethics* Oxford Readings in Philosophy Series (Oxford: Oxford University Press, 2001). Together with Justine C. Burley he has published *A Companion to Genetics: Philosophy and the Genetic Revolution* (Basil Blackwell, Oxford, 2002). He is also the author of *On Cloning* (London: Routledge, 2004).

Arne Ljungqvist graduated as an MD and a PhD from the Medical Faculty, Karolinska Institute, Sweden. Besides his academic career, Ljungqvist distinguished himself in the world of sports, first representing Sweden in the high jump at the Games of the XV Olympiad in Helsinki in 1952, and later as a sports official. He was President of the Swedish Sports Confederation (1989–2001), and is presently Vice-President of the IAAF (1981–), Chairman of the IAAF Medical Commission (1980–), Member of the World Anti-Doping Agency (WADA) since 1989 and Member and Chairman of the Medical Commission of the IOC.

Sigmund Loland is Professor of Sport Philosophy at The Norwegian University of Sport and Physical Education. He has published extensively on topics such as the ethics of sport, sport and ecology, epistemology and movement, and the theory of sport science. His latest book is *Fair Play in Sport: A Moral Norm System* (London: Routledge 2002).

Andy Miah is a Lecturer in Media, Bioethics, and Cyberculture at the University of Paisley, Scotland and a Tutor in the Ethics of Science and Medicine at the Graduate School of Biomedical and Life Sciences, University of Glasgow, Scotland. His research is informed by an applied interest in ethics, technology, and culture, and he has published widely in the areas of cyberculture, sport, and bioethics. He is the author of *Genetically Modified Athletes: Biomedical Ethics, Genes and Sport* (London: Routledge, 2004) and co-editor of *Sport Technology: History, Philosophy and Policy* (Oxford: Elsevier, 2002).

Christian Munthe holds a PhD in practical philosophy and is Associate Professor in the Department of Philosophy, University of Gothenburg, Sweden. His research focuses on ethical issues actualised by the application of gene technology to human beings and the moral assessment of technological risks.

Ingmar Persson is Professor of Practical Philosophy at Gothenburg University, Sweden. He is currently finishing a book, *The Retreat of Reason*, on the rationality of our attitudes to personal identity and free will (forthcoming from Oxford University Press).

Julian Savulescu is Professor and Uehiro Chair in Practical Ethics at the University of Oxford. He established and is Director of the Oxford Centre for Practical Ethics. He was editor of the prestigious *Journal of Medical Ethics*. Julian Savulescu qualified in medicine, bioethics and analytic philosophy. He has published over 100 articles in journals such as the *British Medical Journal*, *The Lancet*, the *Australasian Journal of Philosophy*, *Bioethics*, the *Journal of Medical Ethics*, the *American Journal of Bioethics*, the *Medical Journal of Australia and Philosophy*, and *Psychiatry and Psychology*.

Peter Schjerling is a Senior Researcher at the Copenhagen Muscle Research Centre in Denmark. He studies the basic mechanisms behind the exercise-related activation of muscle genes. He initiated the discussion about gene doping in 1998 and has frequently given interviews to the national and international media on gene doping. He has also been a consultant on the gene doping issue for both the Danish and the Dutch governments and WADA, and is the co-author of an article on the gene doping issue in *Scientific American* (Sept. 2000).

Angela J. Schneider has a PhD in Philosophy in applied ethics. She is an Associate Professor in the School of Kinesiology in the Faculty of Health Sciences at the University of Western Ontario, Canada. Dr Schneider is the former Director of Ethics and Education for the World Anti-Doping Agency and currently conducting her research and supervising graduate students at the International Centre for Olympic Studies. She also won a silver medal for Canada in the 1984 Olympic Games in Los Angeles in the Women's Coxed Fours in Rowing.

Meredith Schwartz is a student finishing the MA program and beginning the PhD program in Philosophy at Dalhousie University, Halifax, Nova Scotia. She holds a Killam Trust Scholarship and a Canadian Institute of Health Research (CIHR) Ethics of Health Research and Policy Doctoral Fellowship. Her first book, *Coping with Choriocarcinoma and Molar Pregnancy* (Your Health Press, Toronto) will be published in 2005.

Susan Sherwin is a Research Fellow in the Department of Philosophy (with cross-appointments to Bioethics, Women's Studies, and Nursing) at Dalhousie University, Halifax, Nova Scotia. She is the author of *No Longer Patient: Feminist Ethics and Health Care* (Philadelphia, PA: Temple University Press, 1992). She has also served as coordinator of the Feminist Health Care Ethics Research Network which jointly published *The Politics of Women's Health: Exploring Agency and Autonomy* (Philadelphia, PA: Temple University Press, 1998). She is a Fellow of the Royal Society of Canada.

Claudio Tamburrini is a Senior Researcher in the Department of Philosophy, Gothenburg University, Sweden. He is the author of *Crime and Punishment?* (Stockholm: Acta Universitatis Stockholmiensis, 1992) and of several international articles on penal philosophy. In the area of the philosophy of sports, he has published *The 'Hand of God'? Essays in the Philosophy of Sports* (Göteborg: Acta Universitatis Gothoburgensis, 2000), which has also been translated into Spanish. In both Sweden and Argentina, Tamburrini's accomplishments include pioneering work in introducing the philosophy of sports as an academic discipline. Together with Torbjön Tännsjö, he is the co-editor of *Values in Sport: Elitism, Nationalism, Gender Equality and the Scientific Manufacture of Winners* (London: E & FN Spon, 2000). At present, he is working on a book on moral relativism and its implications for the punishment of human rights violators. Tamburrini was also a professional soccer player in Argentina.

Torbjörn Tännsjö is Professor of Practical Philosophy at Stockholm University, Sweden. He has published extensively in moral philosophy, political philosophy and bioethics. Together with Claudio Tamburrini, he edited *Values in Sport: Elitism, Nationalism, Gender Equality and the Scientific Manufacture of Winners*

(London: E & FN Spon, 2000). His most recent book is *Understanding Ethics* (Edinburgh: Edinburgh University Press, 2003).

Ivo van Hilvoorde is postdoctoral researcher at the Department of Health Care Ethics and Philosophy, Maastricht University, and at the W.J.H. Mulier Institute, Centre for Research on Sports in Society, 's-Hertogenbosch, the Netherlands. He has published on sport philosophy and educational science. His current work involves the ethics of gene technology in sport and the social-historical emergence of standards and ideals for the fit and sporting body.

Sarah Wilson is a post-doctoral researcher at the Centre for Economic and Social Aspects of Genomics at Lancaster University, currently working with the North West Genetics Knowledge Park. Dr Wilson's particular research interest is in social justice as it relates to issues in bioethics and genetics, and she has recently published several papers on social justice and governance in relation to human genomic databases.

Series editors' preface

This volume is the second contribution by Torbjörn Tännsjö and Claudio Tamburrini to the Ethics and Sport series. It develops many of the themes explored in their earlier volume *Values and Sport* (Routledge, 2000), specifically in the context of contemporary debate and scholarship in genetic ethics and technology. Moreover, it complements the immediately previous book published in the series: Andy Miah's *Genetically Modified Athletes* (Routledge, 2004), whose focus is on the promise and prospects of genetic engineering

The present volume houses disparate voices in the new debate, ranging from optimism to scepticism and dissent. It considers a range of fundamental discussions about the nature of genetic technology and its biochemical basis, and the possibilities for genetic enhancement and genetic testing, moving on to applied areas such as ethical and educational implications, policy critique and, perhaps most importantly, the potential consequences for the configurations of sport itself.

Each of the chapters, by authors already well known in their respective fields, offers critical insight into the challenges of a genetically based re-envisioning of sport and sport sciences. There is little doubt that this book will help to shape the emerging debates in the years to come.

The editors have collected leading voices from both bioethics and the ethics of sport, so that this volume represents a particularly welcome interface between scholars of different sectors of applied ethics. One of the most important functions of this volume, we feel, has been not merely to encourage the confluence of these voices and the richly varied backgrounds their authors draw upon, but also to encourage a genuine and growing collaboration between them.

We hope that the writings of sports ethicists here will contribute to the bioethical tradition in the same way that those of bioethicists have nourished the strongly emerging field of sports ethics.

Mike McNamee, University of Wales, Swansea
Jim Parry, University of Leeds

Introduction

The life sciences and the ethos of sport

Claudio Tamburrini and Torbjörn Tännsjö

Present genetic technology poses a challenge to sport so serious that it is hard to overestimate. What is at stake is the very ethos of sport; nothing less than an epochal confrontation between a model of human identity as spelled out in the Book of Genesis and a science-based libertarian model. According to the former, sports is a means by which we explore human nature, admire it at its peak, and gain self-understanding. It is not up to us to play God or, to put it in a more mundane and secular way, to 'meddle with our evolutionary determined human nature'. According to the latter, secular model, the deliberate adaptation of our biological nature is exactly our prerogative. We have reached a point at last where this prerogative is becoming a genuine possibility. For supporters of the secular model, our destiny is in our own hands. To those of us who do not accept authority, there still exists a deep humanistic obligation: to see to it that our human nature will turn out to be of a kind that is worthy of admiration. And when moulding our biological nature, the sports arena is the perfect place to test out the results of new biological innovations.

It is easy to misrepresent what is now happening within the life sciences and to underestimate the impact it will have on the human condition. Certainly it is true that many prophesies in the field have been premature, in particular when it comes to gene therapy. So now we usually hear the complaint that the biological sciences have been 'hyped' up too much in relation to both health care and to sport. Andy Miah (in Chapter 4) quotes Steve Jones' remark that, 'there is a massive quantity of hype when it comes to gene therapy in sport. I put it in the same ballpark as the babbling nonsense talked about a baldness cure based on gene therapy.' But this adopts a very slippery view of things.

First, even if progress in gene therapy in the life sciences has been slow so far, there is no doubt that there has been progress. So even if we have not yet had to face some of the problems that were envisaged some twenty years ago, we certainly will have to face them in the future, and we cannot exclude the possibility that we will have to face some of them in the near future.

Second, in relation to sport, one of the main complaints against fanciful, science fiction speculation about the future use of gene technology is not well founded. The main complaint is that, in all these prophesies about a future where our human personality has been re-designed, a much too simplistic view of our human genome has been taken for granted.[1] This may well be true of some sorts of speculation but, in relation to sport, this concern is not important. Among the genetic factors explaining success in sport, some seem to be rather simple. This has to do with the fact that sport itself is, in a way, simplistic. In many ways, success is simply a matter of being the strongest, the fastest, and the most focused.

Finally, while it is often claimed that many applications within the health care setting of genetic techniques will be delayed because the techniques cannot be made safe in the foreseeable future, this may well be reason to believe that they will be introduced slowly within the health care setting. However, as Miah also pointed out, sport is different. The idea that if a technique involves unknown risks, it will not be used, is a tricky position to maintain, since individuals can consent to knowing that the risks are uncertain and accept that (unknown) level of risk. Particularly in sport, there are always people who are prepared to take great risks in order to gain only a little in competitive edge. We know this from ordinary doping experiences. And there are nations where the regulation of the relationship between sports and medicine does not conform to the noble aspirations we read about in text books of medical ethics. We are familiar with that phenomenon from the experience of ordinary forms of doping. Considering the difficulties in detecting enhancement achieved through genetic modification, as thoroughly described by Christian Munthe (Chapter 9), we must suspect, therefore, that very soon the first cases of genetically achieved enhancement will appear in the sports arenas. Perhaps they have already made their appearance without announcing their presence.

In this anthology, all the authors take seriously the possibility of genetic enhancement in sports. And an additional theme, of almost the same kind of practical relevance, is the focus of interest of some of the authors: genetic testing and selection of athletes.

OVERVIEW OF THE BOOK

Part I   The state of the art

Part I, 'The state of the art', is devoted to the task of giving an overview of the state of play at present. In Chapter 1 Arne Ljungqvist, Member Chairman of the IOC and the IAAF Medical Commission, puts forward the official stance on genetics in sport, as formulated by the World Anti-doping Agency (WADA). It is interesting to note that the Olympic authorities have not tried to set to one side the problem of gene therapy or genetic testing in sport. Quite to the contrary, these authorities have squarely faced up to the situation in an attempt to be 'ahead of the cheaters'. As reported by Ljungqvist, in 2001 the IOC developed a working group on gene therapy in sport. In 2002 WADA (of which Ljungqvist is Member of the Executive Committee and Board) hosted a meeting to discuss the matter, which led to WADA including a reference to gene doping in their draft 2004 Anti-Doping Code. In its 2005 'List of Prohibited Substances and Methods', WADA makes the following prohibition:

II. PROHIBITED METHODS . . .

M3. GENE DOPING

The non-therapeutic use of cells, genes, genetic elements, or of the modulation of gene expression, having the capacity to enhance athletic performance, is prohibited.[2]

In Chapter 2, Peter Schjerling reviews what can be done at present, and what is likely to become possible in the foreseeable future with respect to genetic modification and testing in sport. While warning us about the potential health risks that genetic technology will bring, the author considers nonetheless the possibility of harm reduction by using the new technique in organised sport teams where physicians are involved.

In Chapter 3, Angela Schneider introduces us to the topics discussed at the Banbury Workshop on Genetic Enhancement of Athletic Performance, New York, organised by WADA in March 2002. Although she is critical of some of the notions included in the conceptual framework of the official anti-doping policy (for instance, the dubious distinction between 'therapy' and 'enhancement'), Schneider nevertheless condones the proscriptive policy defended by Arne Ljungqvist by resorting to the notion of 'public consent', as opposed to the well-established principle of personal consent. In her view, individuals' freedom to undergo a treatment or practice, or a research intervention, does not trump the sport community's right to give or withhold its public consent to methods deemed by it as noxious for the entire practice of sports as a public good.

This part of the anthology is concluded by a chapter by Andy Miah, one of the philosophers of sport who has devoted himself to genetic modification in sport. He notes and welcomes the fact that the Olympic Committee has taken the problem of genetic enhancement and testing seriously, but he questions whether the best approach is to try to 'be ahead of those who cheat'. Perhaps the correct stance to take with respect to the life sciences in sport is rather to try to think through what values are at stake here, before one decides what practical measures to adopt. Rather than just trying to extend existing regulations of doping to genetic techniques, there are good reasons to reflect on the entire problem. According to Miah:

> one might argue that there remains an important question to be asked about the infrastructure of anti-doping. I have attempted to suggest here that this infrastructure must now broaden itself beyond the traditional connections between sports and governments to encompass policy groups concerned with genetic technology more broadly. Without this additional layer of debate and without the broader contextualisation of sport policy about genetics, sports run the risk of marginalising themselves from changing social values about genetic technology. Moreover, they risk developing a policy that is inconsistent with the legal and moral concerns of the genetically modified athlete.

This concern now leads us naturally into Part II, that deals with genetic enhancement of athletes.

Part II   The genetic enhancement of athletes

Part II opens with a chapter written by Torbjörn Tännsjö, who urges us to think about the notion of justice practised in sport. Following on from his argument in 'Is it fascistoid to admire sport heroes?',[3] Tännsjö affirms that the general idea when we contemplate sport is that when all the 'irrelevant' factors have been eliminated, those who win and who therefore receive our admiration are and should be the winners of the genetic lottery. He asks, but what kind of notion of justice renders these people worthy of our admiration? Is it not a strange notion of justice, which allows us to praise people mainly for achievements for which they are not themselves responsible? Does it not come close to the fascistic ideology in this manner to admire mere strength? Does this not run counter to what we think about justice in other fields of our lives? Should we not praise those who have made a free effort to achieve something rather than those who achieved the same thing without having to make any effort of their own?

Based on his critique of the dominant notion about sport justice, Tännsjö claims that once genetic engineering becomes a standard route to athletic success, we have the possibility of returning to a more defensible view of justice in sport. Now we can admire the athlete for the physical constitution he or she has chosen – and we can admire the scientists who made this possible through their marvellous inventions. So rather than banning the introduction of genetic enhancement in sport, we ought to welcome such a development, he claims. The genetic design of winners means that we can watch sports competitions without the uneasy feeling that, when we cheer for the winners, we reveal our inclination towards any fascist ideology.

This attack upon the standard notion of justice in sport does not go unchallenged, of course. In the following chapter, Tännsjö's philosopher colleague, Ingmar Persson, claims that the contrast between sport and other areas of our lives drawn by Tännsjö is spurious. The kind of admiration for the winners that we express when we watch sport is no different from, neither better nor worse than, what takes place, for example, in the sciences and in the arts. Thus the rationale put forward by Tännsjö for accepting genetic enhancement in sport is not well grounded. This is not, of course, to say that genetic enhancement in sport should be banned. In the present context, Persson does not himself take up any stance on this question.

Tännsjö's position that there are good reasons to welcome genetic enhancement in sport is a radical one, of course. Most of the discussion in relation to genetic modification of athletes has focused rather on the arguments *against* allowing genetic enhancement. Our authors have taken it for granted that there is a strong incentive among both athletes and scientists to enter this field and the question raised has been: what is so terrible about genetic modification?

One argument why genetic modification should not be allowed has been that it threatens the autonomy or dignity of those who become subject to modification.

This line of argument has been taken up in particular with respect to germline genetic modification, i.e. with respect to genetic modification of germ cells or early embryos, where the effects are inherited by the offspring of the individual who has the modification. Tännsjö attempts to rebut these arguments in general and in the context of sport, in particular. They are also taken up by Claudio Tamburrini in Chapter 7, according to whom these arguments are flawed. Rather than restraining the autonomy of a person, germline genetic modifications might offer the modified person a rich(er) repertoire of traits of personality to develop. Thus, parents' commitment to this new technique enhances, rather than restrains, the very capacity for autonomy of their child. For it is certainly up to the child him or herself to decide what characteristics to develop in life. Germline genetic enhancement, Tamburrini claims, is not essentially different from the ordinary education of children.

Tamburrini's argument is scrutinised in the following chapter, written by Ivo van Hilvoorde, who admits that germline genetic enhancement need not as such restrict the autonomy of the person who undergoes it. And yet, germline genetic enhancement is deeply problematic, according to van Hilvoorde. The problem with germline genetic enhancement, rather than with the technique as such, relates to the kind of intentions behind the parental decision to resort to it. According to van Hilvoorde, the attempt to mould the biological nature of one's child is, notwithstanding Tamburrini's arguments, at variance with a decent and quite natural impulse to educate one's child.

Part III Genetic testing of athletes

Part III starts with Chapter 9 by Christian Munthe,[4] where he addresses the control programmes necessary to detect athletes' illegitimate uses of genetic technology and relates them to several ethical issues familiar within the field of genetic testing for health purposes. In particular, he discusses the questions of how to handle and communicate information about athletes' health uncovered by the testing, and what hardships – caused by the testing itself – one can reasonably require athletes to endure.

In Chapter 10, Ruth Chadwick discusses nutrigenomics applied to effectiveness of diet with reference to sport. As Aristotle recognised, what is appropriate food for one athlete may not be appropriate for another person not devoted to the practice of sport. 'Functional food' would presumably be regarded as preferable to the taking of a banned drug, although it might have the same effect. Thus, the author believes, given the increasing medicalisation of nutrition, and 'in so far as the dividing line between food and drugs is undermined, we may need to revisit the ways in which at society level we deal with the conceptual and regulatory issues around the boundary between food and drugs, and the use of such foods in competition'.

In Chapter 11, Julian Savulescu examines the ethical implications of the genetic testing of boxers to identify those who are most exposed to brain damage as a consequence of repeatedly being hit during fights. Recent research suggests that a major risk factor for chronic traumatic brain injury in boxers is the presence of the APOEe4 allele (an apolipoprotein which predisposes the elderly to develop Alzheimer's disease). In his chapter Savulescu raises the question of whether testing to identify those boxers who carry two copies of APOEe4 should be made compulsory and whether those most at risk should be prevented from boxing.

Part IV   Genetic technology and the ethos of sport

Much of the opposition to using genetic technologies in sports comes from the fear that this will alter the very nature of sport. Some people even picture a future scenario in which elite sports become simply show business. If such a sport world turns into reality, are there sport disciplines that are more vulnerable to the effects of the new genetic technology? And will they become less attractive for the public? These questions are addressed in Part IV.

In Chapter 12, Lincoln Allison contrasts two different sport traditions, which he calls 'athleticism' and 'sportmanism'. The former sees performance as an end in itself, while, for the latter, performance is merely incidental to the ethical and social value implicit in sport. According to this author, bio-chemical and particularly bio-technical enhancements will sharpen the tensions between these two traditions. This, he argues, will lead to a decline in the disciplines that belong in the 'athleticist' tradition (such as swimming, cycling and track and field) at an elite level while, on the other hand, will lead to an improved market for sports where judgement, tactics, skill and teamwork are at a premium (such as soccer, basketball and cricket).

In Chapter 13, Sigmund Loland argues that the cause of the doping problem (either chemical or genetic) is to be found at the systemic level of highly specialised sport performances. Starting with an examination of the basic elements of an athletic performance to more precisely define what is meant by 'specialisation', this author formulates what he calls 'the vulnerability thesis'. In short, his thesis runs as follows: the higher the degree of specialisation of performance in a given sport, the more vulnerable it becomes to the use of gene-technological means of performance enhancement.

This part of the book concludes with Gunnar Breivik's discussion of central aspects of the ideological foundation of modern elite sports. In Chapter 14, he attempts to show that doping is a natural extension of elite sport and not an accidental development. Starting from how doping has been defined, he goes on to sketch the new genetic techniques, the new ethical problems they create and their implications for human identity, autonomy and dignity.

Part V   Gender equality and gene technology in sport

Roughly speaking, feminist thinking comes in two radically different varieties. On the one hand, there is a gender-blind egalitarian version of feminist thought, dating back to Plato, Woolstonecraft, and J.S. Mill, stressing that, essentially, men and women are no different. Crucially, then, the feminist project means treating equals equally. The most radical expression of this idea is certainly Sulamith Firestone,[5] who defends the idea that artificial wombs should be welcomed, ascertaining that women and men can share responsibility equally, not only of child rearing, but also of child bearing. On the other hand, there is a feminist tradition which stresses gender specificity: that men and women are essentially different. A just treatment of men and women, then, means that these differences are taken properly into account.[6] The idea that the sexes are essentially different is traditionally associated with sexual prejudice. Recently, it has been taken up by some feminist thinkers. Within the sport context these differences between the two traditions become conspicuously clear. In Chapter 15, Tamburrini and Tännsjö defend the gender-blind egalitarian position. Building on previous work, they argue that men and women should be allowed to compete on equal terms against each other in sport.[7] Individuals have different talents for achievements in sport, and even though statistical correlations between sex and sporting performance actually exist, they argue that sex as such is not directly relevant to success. Rather, besides mental capabilities, what determines the winner in a sports competition are certain physical characteristics, such as weight, length, muscular mass, and so forth. So, if we want to make distinctions within sport in order to render the outcome of competition less predictable, we should focus on these characteristics themselves rather than simply on sex, as is typically the case in sport competitions at present.

One problem with this position is that, eventually, it may turn out that in some sports, there are some men who, it is true, can rather easily defeat any woman. And it may turn out that, in the most prestigious (weight, length, muscular mass, and so forth) classes, only men appear and excel. If this is so and, if this is conceived of as a problem, then, the authors claim, genetic engineering may provide a solution to it. Provided the conjecture is true that it is easier, through genetic engineering, for those who lag behind to catch up with those who are ahead than for those who are already ahead to move even further on, genetic engineering may allow some women – whom they call the Bio-Amazons – to become as strong as the strongest men.

This proposal has raised severe criticism from many renowned bioethicists and philosophers of sport, included in this volume. It seems that they are prepared to take up some kind of gender essentialist feminist position with respect to sport. In Chapter 16, Susan Sherwin and Meredith Schwarz write that

> the principal problem with equating equality with sameness is that it fails to question the standards as they are currently set. Requiring oppressed groups to be the same as dominant groups in order to be given equal respect creates a double-bind because the group is usually oppressed on the very basis of some difference, e.g., gender, skin color, sexual orientation, or (dis)ability.

They refer to women's tennis as an example where different (feminine) skills are required rather than male ones (as in men's tennis).

In Chapter 17, Ruth Chadwick and Sarah Wilson claim that there are alternatives to the Bio-Amazons 'project'. An alternative to the creation of the

Bio-Amazons could be creating a reward structure in order to bring gender equality into sport. Finally, in Chapter 18, Simona Giordano and John Harris go even further in their repudiation of the egalitarian argument put forward by the editors which is, they claim, 'in fact discriminatory, and reveal[s] a male chauvinist ideology'. This means, however, interestingly enough, but not unexpectedly, that some of these authors have to question elitist sport as such.

We have come full circle, then, and we are back to where this volume started, with a critical examination of the peculiar notion of justice inherent in the ethos of sport. If we are interested in equality, Giordano and Harris claim, we should 'promote sports and physical activities in larger strata of population' and 'discuss ways in which everybody – regardless of sex, age, ethnic or social background – could be enabled to participate in sports, exercise and physical activities.'

This is not the place for us, the editors of this volume, to decide on these matters. We believe, however, that the last word has not being said on the issue of gender equality in sports or, for that matter, on the further questions related to genetic enhancement addressed in this volume. Genetic technology has already made its mark on general medicine. Probably, it will relatively soon be applied in sport medicine as well. Radical and profound changes in the way we have regarded phenomena such as, for instance, curing and enhancing, privacy and consent in testing procedures, autonomy, fairness in competition and related ideas of sports and even the very notion of male and female, are facing us at present. Confronted with this reality, the challenge posed to both scholars and the public is to find a way to assert the specifically human in the highly technified sporting practices we embark on today. To do that, we need to renounce preconceived notions and provide ourselves with an open, searching attitude to deal with current developments in the new sciences. Particularly, a critical and bold debate is indispensable. It is the aim of the editors that this book will be received as a worthy contribution to that debate.

NOTES

1   In a position paper drafted by the Council for Responsible Genetics in 1992, it stated that:

> Inserting new segments of DNA into the germline could have major, unpredictable consequences for both the individual and the future of the species that include the introduction of susceptibilities to cancer and other disease into the human gene pool.

Germline modifications, in other words, have little practical appeal but generate considerable health risks for the species and ethical apprehension. Quoted in Ted Peters, *Playing God? Genetic Determinism and Human Freedom*, 2nd edn (London: Routledge, 2003), Chapter 6: 'The Question of Germ Line Intervention', p. 151.

2   See http://www.wada-ama.org/rtecontent/document/list_2005.pdf.

3   Included in a previous volume in this series, *Values in Sport: Elitism, Nationalism, Gender Equality and the Scientific Manufacture of Winners*, T. Tännsjö and C. M. Tamburrini, (eds) (London: E & FN Spon, 2000), pp. 24–38.

4   Munthe has previously written a seminal article on the impact of genetic technology in the field of elite sports. See his 'Selected Champions: Making Winners in the Age of Genetic Technology', included in Tännsjö and Tamburrini, op. cit., pp. 217–21.

5   See her book *The Dialectic of Sex* (New York: Bantam, 1971).

6   See, for example, Martha Minnow, *Making All the Difference: Inclusion, Exclusion, and American Law* (Ithaca, NY: Cornell University Press, 1990); Gisela Bock and Susan James, (eds) *Beyond Equality and Difference: Citizenship, Feminist Politics, and Female Subjectivity* (London: Routledge, 1992); Christine A. Littleton, 'Reconstructing Sexual Equality', *California Law Review*, 1987, 75(4): 1279–335; and Joan W. Scott, 'Deconstructing Equality-Versus-Difference', *Feminist Studies*, 1988, 14(1): 35–50.

7   See T. Tännsjö, 'Against Sexual Discrimination in Sports', in Tännsjö and Tamburrini, op. cit., pp. 101–15, and C. Tamburrini, 'The Return of the Amazons', in *The 'Hand of God'? Essays in the Philosophy of Sport* (Göteborg: Acta Universitatis Gothoburgensis), 2000, Chapter 6, pp. 104–47.

Part I

The state of the art

1 The international anti-doping policy and its implementation

Arne Ljungqvist

INTRODUCTION

Although the use of performance-enhancing drugs in competitive sport has a long history, the incident at the Olympic Games in Rome 1960 marks the starting point of the modern fight against doping. At those Games a Danish cyclist collapsed during the 100km team race and later died in hospital. He had received a stimulating drug before the race. The drug in combination with the extreme heat during the competition probably caused his collapse and death. The Rome Games were the first Olympic Games to be televised world-wide. To have a drug-related death of an Olympic competitor exposed to the world was too much for the International Olympic Committee (IOC). Thus, the IOC created a 'Medical Commission' (IOC MC) which was asked to propose an action plan to combat the use of drugs in Olympic Sport (Dirix and Sturbois, 1998).

IOC MC: THE EARLY YEARS

The IOC MC recruited eminent scientists in the field of research in stimulating drugs and drug analysis. At that time stimulants of various kinds were the drugs known to be used in sport for the purpose of performance enhancement. The IOC MC listed those drugs that they felt should be prohibited, worked out methods for their detection and designed rules and regulations to be applied during the Olympic Games. The IOC endorsed the proposals presented to them by the IOC MC, and tentative doping controls were carried out during the Olympic Games in 1964. This control programme was expanded at the Games in 1968, and in Munich in 1972 large numbers of doping controls for various types of stimulants were conducted. That is also when one of the first controversial cases occurred. The American gold medallist in the 400m freestyle swim, 16-year-old Rick Demont, was disqualified and deprived of his gold medal following a positive doping test for ephedrine. He had reported that he was using the medication for the treatment of his asthma, but that did not help. Ephedrine was prohibited – finished! There was no mechanism in place at the time to apply for exemption to use a prohibited substance because of medical need.

The IOC MC soon discovered that not only stimulants were being misused in sport. Also anabolic steroids were widely used. It appeared that they had come into sport in the late 1950s or early 1960s but the sport world had been unprepared to deal with the situation at the time. The IOC MC now had to cope with a totally new problem. Steroids were taken during training in order to enhance muscular growth and strength. Doping controls limited to competitions would be ineffective since steroid takers would only have to stop taking the drugs some time before the competitions in order to test negative, and yet benefit from their effects. Moreover, there were no analytical methods available for their detection. Thus, analytical procedures were worked out and new rules for 'out-of-competition testing' were introduced. It proved very difficult, however, to introduce proper out-of-competition testing without interfering with the athletes' right to privacy. Not even today is there a sufficiently extensive out-of-competition testing programme in place internationally. And it has proven particularly difficult to implement an international programme of completely unannounced out-of-competition testing. That was one of many reasons for the creation of the World Anti-Doping Agency (WADA) in 1999.

THE MODERN ERA

Although the official standpoint of the IOC was to combat doping by all available means, the attitude among the International Federations and many countries was more relaxed. It later came out that there even existed sophisticated and state-run doping programmes in order to produce top international athletes, e.g. in the former GDR (Berendonk, 1991). At the Olympic Games in Seoul 1988, however, something happened that made the world wake up. 'The best athlete in the world' (i.e. the winner of the men's 100 meters final, Ben Johnson) was found to be doped with steroids. Not only had he won a spectacular race – he had also broken the world record. Sport stood at a crossroad and had to choose the future strategy. The decision was not to give in, but to step up the fight against doping.

The sporting world united in the fight against doping after the Ben Johnson scandal. The collapse of the 'Iron Curtain' followed by the revelations about the state-run doping programme in the GDR further helped to unify the international sport in that fight. Doping was seen as a deadly threat to competitive sport. The goal was to eradicate all doping in sport. The fourcorner stones of the anti-doping strategy should be strengthened: information, education, doping controls and research. As a consequence, international cooperation in anti-doping activities expanded through bilateral and multilateral agreements, and new national anti-doping agencies were created (Houlihan, 1999). In Sweden the national Sports Confederation had already made it clear a long time ago that doping was unacceptable, and the government had put extra resources at their disposal for an efficient fight against doping. Now that policy had reached the international level.

It was ironic that the case of a track and field athlete should make the world wake up to doping. The world governing body of Track and Field Athletics (the IAAF) had actually been the leading international federation in the fight against doping for many years. Although the IOC MC had undertaken pioneering work, the IOC alone have the responsibility for the Olympic Games. The international federations, on the other hand, are responsible for the year-round activities in their sports.

Thus, the IAAF soon recognized the need for having scientifically safe procedures in place for the analysis of doping control samples. A programme for the 'accreditation' of doping laboratories was developed in the mid-1970s. Once fully developed the programme was transferred to the IOC in 1983 in order to encourage other sports to conduct doping controls and make use of competent laboratories. The IAAF was also the first federation to test for anabolic steroids, which happened at the European Championships in Rome in 1974. The IOC followed at the Olympic Games two years later. Furthermore, the IAAF was the first international federation to introduce unannounced out-of-competition doping controls in the early 1990s. The programme was based on the experience of the Swedish out-of-competition control programme that had been introduced some ten years earlier.

Following the Ben Johnson scandal, sports authorities tried to catch up with the development in doping. The misused substances were identified and the 'doping list' was accordingly amended and increased. More laboratories became accredited. The attempts to develop analytical methods for new drugs were intensified, although resources for research remained poor. Education programmes were developed in many countries and by international federations. Some countries even introduced national legislation against doping, e.g. Sweden in 1992.

LEGAL ASPECTS

One fundamental principle of the anti-doping policy is to protect all those athletes who do not take performance-enhancing drugs from having to compete against those who do. Although preventive information and education measures are important, they are not enough. To make sure by doping controls that the rules are observed is, therefore, an indispensable part of any anti-doping programme. Should an athlete test positive, however, he/she is only suspected of having committed a doping offence until he/she has been offered a hearing and a final decision has been taken. Any athlete under suspicion must have his/her right guaranteed in accordance with basic human rights principles. This also includes the possibility for the athlete to appeal against any decision that may be taken against him/her. To that effect the IAAF was the first international sports organization to establish a Court of Arbitration in 1982 (Tarasti, 2000). In 1983 the IOC took a similar decision and established the 'Court of Arbitration for Sport' (CAS) in Lausanne. Again, the IAAF was the pioneer.

As the fight against doping became more intense, increasing numbers of athletes were found to be doped. Since such athletes will have their reputation ruined and in many instances also lose their main income, they tend to flatly deny having used doping substances. This has opened up a new market for lawyers as defenders of such athletes, particularly so in the United States. Of course, the athlete under suspicion does have his/her right to a proper defence safeguarded, as explained above, but the ever increasing legal fights tend to become too costly.

The case of the former world record holder in 400m running, Harry 'Butch' Reynolds, is a relevant example. He was found doped with steroids in 1990, a fact which was finally established by the IAAF Court of Arbitration, albeit he strongly denied it. Reynolds then appealed to a District Court in his US home state Ohio, which decided that Reynolds was not doped and that the IAAF should pay him US$27 million to compensate for his loss of income and reputation. Although the IAAF maintained that the District Court had no jurisdiction in the case, they had to appeal to the next level in the USA, the Circuit Appeals Court. Had the IAAF not done so, all their assets in the USA would have remained frozen (Mobil Oil was then the main IAAF sponsor). The Appeals Court overturned the decision by the District Court. Reynolds then appealed to the Supreme Court which dismissed his appeal. Thus, the IAAF finally won the case after four years, but at great costs for both Reynolds and the IAAF.

One further, and dramatic, example is the former British Athletic Federation. They wrongfully declared an athlete doped in the mid-1990s, following which legal costs and compensation to the athlete made the federation go bankrupt.

As legal cases have become more common, the discrepancies in doping regulations between international federations, and even nations, have been identified as a considerable problem. The same doping offence can result in different sanctions depending upon the sport and the nationality of the athlete. The need for harmonized rules became apparent. But this could not be achieved by the sports movement alone. The IOC, therefore, organized a 'World Conference on Doping' in Lausanne in February 1999 with the aim of achieving harmonization of Anti-Doping rules across the world of sports (Lausanne Declaration, 1999). The Lausanne Declaration was adopted by the IOC Executive Board in March and resulted in the creation of the 'World Anti-Doping Agency' (WADA). Half of the WADA Board is composed of representatives of the sports movement (athletes and leaders) and the other half is composed of representatives of governments around the world. It was agreed that the activities of WADA should be financed half by the Olympic movement and half by the governments.

WADA

Soon after its inception WADA started to develop a 'Strategic Plan'. There it stated that doping is unacceptable and should be eradicated because it is against the spirit of sport, against medical ethics and can be dangerous to the health of the athletes. As a representative of the sports movement on the Board of WADA, I found the attitude of the governmental representatives particularly interesting. They unanimously and openly declared a 'zero tolerance' policy with respect to doping.

WADA slowly started to became operational in 2000. The four main tasks were:

1 To harmonize the doping rules for all sports under a 'World Anti-Doping Code'.
2 To initiate out-of-competition doping controls in sports organizations and geographical areas where those did not exist.
3 To produce information and education material.
4 To fund research in anti-doping with particular emphasis on the development of scientifically safe methods for the detection of existing and future doping substances and methods.

From time to time the idea emerges in the general debate in society that it would be just as good, or even recommended, to let doping be allowed. It should then be noted that such an idea has no support whatsoever in the sports community, the political community or the medical community. It is also totally rejected by those who have the greatest interest, namely the athletes themselves. Thus the ultimate goal of WADA is the eradication of all doping in sport.

THE FUTURE

When the modern fight against doping started there was a huge gap between those who doped, or wished to dope, and those who tried to stop it. Although the IOC had taken action in the early 1960s, too many international federations and countries remained inactive. The Ben Johnson scandal and the collapse of the Iron Curtain changed that situation. Through joint efforts, the fight has now become more aggressive and successful. A recent example was the finding of Nesp in three cross-country skiers at the Olympic Winter Games in Salt Lake City in 2002. Nesp can be considered an 'artificial' erythropoitein that promotes the production of red blood corpuscles and thereby the oxygen delivery to body tissues, which is of importance in endurance events. The drug had been on the market for a few months only, but methods for its detection had already been developed. This is a lesson to be learnt, the next challenge probably being the misuse of gene transfer technology in sport ('gene doping').

In order not to fall behind again, WADA organized an expert workshop on 'Gene Doping' at Banbury Center in Cold Spring Harbor, New York, in March 2002. The aim was to establish 'the state of art' in gene therapy and discuss the potential risk of its future misuse in elite sport. Experts from different parts of the world in the fields of genetics, gene therapy, biochemistry, physiology, cell biology, sports medicine, ethics and law gathered there. Among the many conclusions reached, it is worth mentioning: (1) there was judged to be an obvious risk that future progress in gene therapy research may be misused in sport: (2) such misuse should be prohibited since it will be against medical ethics as well as sports ethics, and would be dangerous to the health of the athlete; and (3) funding should be directed towards the development of methods for the detection of such misuse; the difficulties in developing such methods were recognized but judged not to be insurmountable. WADA has already started to fund research in this area.

'Gene doping' was included in the IOC list of banned substances and methods for 2003 and its prohibition also appears in the 'World Anti-Doping Code' which is intended to become operational as from the Olympic Games in Athens 2004 (World Anti-Doping Code, Montreal, 2003).

CONCLUSION

Virtually all doping substances are medicines, most of them obtainable only on prescription. They are intended for the prevention or cure of disease or alleviation of disease-related symptoms. Their administration to healthy young people is against basic pharmacotherapeutical principles and represents, therefore, medical malpractice.

The modern fight against drug misuse in sport has a history of about forty years. At the start, those who doped were far ahead of those who tried to stop such practice. As the international fight has become more coordinated and intense, the gap has diminished. Today the gap has virtually disappeared, a recent example being the finding of Nesp in three skiers at the Salt Lake City Olympic Games in 2002. Nesp is an 'artificial' erythropoietin that had then been on the market for only a few months, yet there was a method ready to test for it.

The creation of WADA in 1999 is a joint effort by the international sports movement and governments around the world to eradicate doping from sport. It reflects a common attitude that doping is unacceptable because it is against the spirit of sport, against medical ethics and can be dangerous to the health of the athletes.

The strongest pressure group for an intensified fight against doping is the athletes themselves, as expressed in several statements by the athletes commissions of international sports federations and by the Athletes Commission of the International Olympic Committee.

REFERENCES

Berendonk, B. (1991) *Doping-Dokumente: Von der Forschung zum Betrug*. Berlin: Springer-Verlag.

Dirix, A. and Sturbois, X. (1998) *The First Thirty Years of the International Olympic Committee Medical Commission*. Lausanne: The International Olympic Committee.

Houlihan, B. (1999) *Dying to Win: Doping in Sport and the Development of Anti-Doping Policy*. 2nd edn. Strasbourg: Council of Europe.

Lausanne Declaration, (1999) *Olympic Review*, XXVI-25: 17–18.

Tarasti, L. (2000) *Legal Solutions in International Doping Cases: Awards by the IAAF Arbitration Panel 1985–1999*. Milan: SEP Editrice.

WADA (2003) *World Anti-Doping Code*. Montreal: World Anti-Doping Agency.

2 The basics of gene doping

Peter Schjerling

WHAT IS GENE DOPING?

Gene doping is doping based on gene therapy which is a medical treatment involving the use of gene modification in the patients. That is, gene therapy is adding or altering genes in cells within the body in order to treat a disease. Gene therapy is still at the experimental state, but its potential is very high. As with normal medical treatment, some treatments can have a beneficial effect on the performance of athletes and can therefore be expected to be used as doping.

At present, gene doping is most likely not in use, but the fear is that when gene therapy develops, it will create a huge potential for doping that will have a high impact on athletic performance and be virtually impossible to detect (McCrory, 2003). Therefore, in 1998 a discussion was initiated on how to deal with this potential threat to the sports society (Hundevadt, 1998). This concern has been taken up by the World Anti-Doping Agency (WADA) and since 2003 gene doping has been placed on the official doping list (www.wada-ama.org).

This chapter will give an overview of gene doping and provide some idea about the potential in gene doping.

WHAT IS A GENE?

Our hereditary material is our deoxyribonucleic adic (DNA), which contains the blueprint for building the organism. DNA is very long stretches of the four building blocks: A, C, T, and G. The order (sequence) of these four 'letters' determines the DNA codes, as the order of our normal 26 letters in the alphabet determines what this text is about. The human DNA consists of about $3 \square 10 9$ such letters that can be subdivided into about 30,000 genes. Each gene is a region of the DNA containing the blueprint for a specific protein. Whereas the DNA/gene contains the information, the protein provides the function. Some proteins, like the collagens, are responsible for the structure of the body, whereas others, the enzymes, catalyze the various processes within the body, such as the conversion of sugar to energy. Many proteins, in fact, just regulate the production of other proteins, either within the same cell (e.g. transcription factors) or in other cells (hormones).

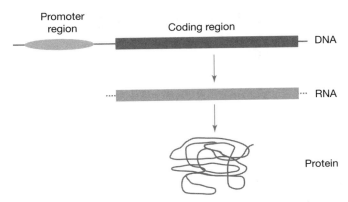

Figure 2.1 From the gene to the protein. The gene consists of a coding region and a regulatory region, the promoter. When the promoter is activated, a transcript is made of the coding region, the RNA, which is then decoded by the machinery of the cell to produce protein.

Each gene consists of a coding sequence preceded by a regulatory sequence termed a promoter (Figure 2.1). The coding sequence contains the actual blueprint used by the machinery of the cell to produce the specific protein, whereas the promoter determines when and how much should be produced. By the binding of different regulatory proteins (transcription factors) to the promoter sequence, the activity of the gene is regulated. When the gene is activated, then a transcript (copy) is made of the coding region (RNA) which is then transported to the protein synthesis complex. By reading the four-letter code in the RNA, a specific protein is made. The amount of protein made is a function of the amount of RNA that is produced which in turn is a function of the activity of the gene.

HOW TO MODIFY GENES

Since the amount of protein produced is a function of the activity of the gene, more of a specific protein can be produced by modifying the regulation of the gene encoding the protein. Since the coding region of the gene contains the blueprint for the protein, the simplest way is to take out the coding region and then add another, more active, regulatory region. This is very simple to do in a laboratory by cutting out the DNA of interest (the coding region) and then sticking it together with the new regulatory DNA. The new gene can then be inserted into a vector which allows the DNA to be amplified in bacterial cells or into a virus which allows the DNA to be amplified in cell cultures. After amplification, the DNA can then be purified and introduced into the body.

HOW TO INSERT THE NEW ARTIFICIAL GENES

After the artificial, more active, gene has been constructed in the laboratory, it has to be introduced into the cells of the body. There are three different ways to achieve this:

1   Injection of the DNA directly into the body. A few cell types in the body are able to take up the DNA directly, especially the muscle cells. So by simply injecting the DNA into a muscle, some muscle cells will acquire the new artificial gene and start to produce the protein of interest.
2   First, introduce the new gene to cells in the laboratory and then inject these cells into the body. Cells can be removed from the body and cultured in the laboratory where the artificial DNA can then be introduced. The modified cells can then be reintroduced into the body.
3   Infection with a virus modified to carry the new gene. The most efficient way, however, is to let nature do the job. Viruses are essentially just micro needles capable of introducing foreign DNA (the virus DNA) into cells. By replacing the virus's own DNA with the artificial DNA, these new viruses can then be used to infect the subject. The modified virus will then introduce the DNA into the cells of the body.

The direct injection is simple but also very inefficient and limited to a few specific cell types. The use of a virus, on the other hand, is much more efficient but since all kinds of cell types will receive the artificial DNA, this also increases the likelihood of unwanted side effects. The most controllable is by far the use of cells modified in the laboratory. However, this method is relatively complicated, inefficient and limited to cell types, like muscle cells, that can be taken out and reintroduced.

REGULATION OF GENES

Until recently most artificial genes used for gene therapy tests simply had a permanently active promoter in front of the coding region for the protein of interest. In this approach the amount of protein produced is simply a function of the efficiency of insertion of the gene into the body. However, for most proteins, especially the hormones, too much production can be very problematic. Therefore, a better approach is to use a promoter for which the activity can be regulated. To construct a regulatable promoter for use in humans has proved difficult. But, in recent years different regulatory systems have been adapted that can do the trick. These promoters respond to different kinds of drugs, e.g. antibiotics and hormones that can be given to the patients to activate the artificial gene (Agha-Mohammadi and Lotze, 2000). These promoters are still in their infancy, but demonstrate that it can be done.

HOW LONG DOES THE MODIFICATION LAST?

When the artificial gene successfully gets into the cell, the DNA is stable and in principle the new gene will be there forever. However, if the cell starts to divide, then the exact nature of the insertion becomes important. The artificial DNA is not able to replicate, so unless it is integrated into the genomic DNA, the artificial DNA will not replicate and therefore only one of the daughter cells will acquire the artificial DNA. Since dividing cells also will die, to keep the number of cells in the body constant, non-replicating DNA will eventually get lost with a speed depending on the turnover time of the cell type. However, not all cell types divide in an adult body. Especially interesting in the present context are the muscle fibres, which are multinucleated cells that relatively easily take up the artificial DNA and never divide.

In a very small fraction of the cells the DNA will by chance integrate into the genomic DNA, in which case the artificial DNA will be replicated and all daughter cells will possess the new gene. Therefore, the artificial gene will not be lost over time. In most cases, when viruses are used to introduce the DNA, the virus system actually causes the DNA to be integrated into the genome and therefore the integration is stable.

Whether or not the DNA happens to be integrated into the genome, the immune system plays an even more important role in determining the survival time of the artificial DNA. To facilitate the work with the artificial DNA, specific bacterial or virus DNA sequences (a vector sequence) are added to the artificial gene. In many cases this will activate the immune system which will then kill the cells that have acquired the artificial DNA. In some cases the cells will be killed within a few days, but often within months.

Since gene therapy is a new field, no long-term tests have yet been carried out, but with the right system there is no reason to believe that the modification cannot last for the entire life of the subject. Although for most types of gene therapy the long-lasting effect is the goal, for some treatments it would be preferable for the artificial DNA to have a short survival time, e.g. healing of injuries. Furthermore, unlike with normal medication, gene therapy does not readily offer the possibility of terminating the treatment if problems arise. Once the artificial DNA is inside the body, it cannot be removed. However, methods are underway to try to overcome this problem by including an emergency gene that, upon administration of a specific drug, will kill the modified cells or alternatively remove the modified DNA (Siprashvili and Khavari, 2004).

THE POSSIBILITIES TODAY

In the early phase gene doping cases will probably be the direct abuse of treatments already developed for gene therapy. Below are some illustrative examples of gene therapy experiments which have the potential for gene doping.

EPO

Erythropoietin (EPO) is a potent hormone for regulating the amount of oxygen-carrying red blood cells in the blood. The blood volume percentage of red blood cells (hematocrit) is tightly regulated by EPO, which is produced in the kidneys. Since the hematocrit level is very important in endurance performance, EPO has received a great deal of focus in doping. The use of EPO requires injections several times a week to sustain an increased hematocrit level. In a few weeks after cessation of the EPO, the hematocrit level will return to normal.

One of the major problems for patients with kidney failure is the lack of EPO production, which cause anemia. In the past fifteen years it has been possible to treat these patients with EPO but the treatment is very expensive and requires injections several times a week. Therefore, EPO has received much attention as a good candidate for gene therapy for several years.

In 1994, Tripathy *et al.* demonstrated in mice that one single injection with a virus delivering an activated EPO gene increased the hematocrit level from the normal 48 per cent to 70 per cent for at least four months (Tripathy *et al.* 1994). Later similar experiments were performed in monkeys, where the hematocrit level was raised from the normal 40 per cent to 60–70 per cent for at least six months (Svensson *et al.*, 1997; Zhou *et al.*, 1998) (Figure 2.2).

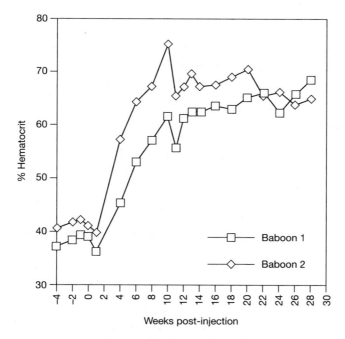

Figure 2.2 Hematocrit level in two monkeys after a single injection with a virus containing an artificial EPO gene. Reprinted from Zhou S., Murphy J. E., Escobedo J. A., Dwarki V. J. (*Gene Therapy*) 5, 665–70 (1998), with permission from Nature.

These experiments demonstrated the potential of gene therapy in that this huge effect lasted for many months after just one single injection. Presumably they can last even longer but the experiments were terminated. However, they also illustrated the current weakness of gene therapy, namely that the level of production cannot easily be controlled. A hematocrit level of 60 per cent will increase the viscosity of the blood to dangerously high levels and therefore, very likely, will cause heart failure.

The success of EPO production has led to many experiments with regulatory promoters to try to gain control over the EPO production (Bohl *et al.*, 1998; Ye *et al.*, 1999; Rizzuto *et al.*, 1999; Terada *et al.*, 2002; Nordstrom 2003; Siprashvili and Khavari, 2004). These regulatory systems all used engineered promoters that are responsive to different kinds of drugs such as the antibiotic tetracycline and the abortion drug mifeprestrone. To achieve this, another artificial gene is included that produces a protein responsive to the drug. In the presence of the drug, this protein will then activate the promoter of the artificial EPO gene. Recent reports have shown in mice and rat models that such a regulated system can be used to treat anemia (Ataka *et al.*, 2003; Johnston *et al.*, 2003).

IGF-1 and myostatin

Whereas EPO gene therapy has a high potential for abuse in endurance type sports, there is not yet any obvious gene therapy targets that would be useful in strength-dependent sports. The normal use of anabolic steroids is not easily transferable to gene therapy since steroids are not proteins and therefore are not directly produced from a gene. Instead they are produced by the conversion of other substances with different enzymes (proteins). To produce anabolic steroids by gene therapy, it would therefore be necessary to include several different genes in a coordinated fashion. At present this is still too complicated but might be possible in the future.

Nevertheless, some interesting genes can be found that might be useful in strength-dependent sports, but since they currently do not receive much interest as potential drugs in normal gene therapy the development of functional constructs is limited. Insulin-like growth factor 1 (IGF-1) and myostatin are such potential candidates. IGF-1 is a growth factor for many organs in the body and localized production of IGF-1 in an organ can induce growth of the specific organ. So, by taking the IGF-1 coding region, fusing it with an active promoter and injecting the gene into a muscle Barton-Davis *et al.* demonstrated in mice that the muscle then grows and increases in strength (Barton-Davis *et al.*, 1998). Myostatin, on the other hand, is a negative regulator of muscle growth. By inactivating the gene entirely in mice (knock-out mice) a supermouse was generated with enormous muscles (McPherron *et al.*, 1997) (Figure 2.3). These mice have in fact been given the nickname 'Schwarzenegger mice'. Inactivation of the myostatin production requires that the gene is inactivated in most cells, which is not currently possible in the adult human body. Instead factors interfering with myostatin function could be used. Inhibition of the normal myostatin function has been accomplished by

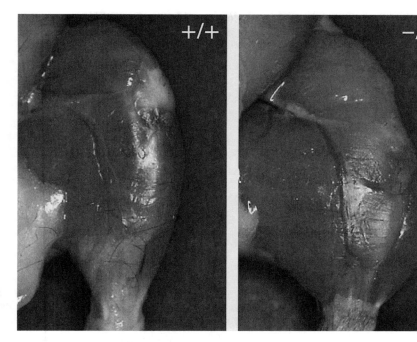

Figure 2.3 Inactivation of the myostatin gene. The left picture shows the front leg of a normal mouse and the right picture the front leg of a mouse with the myostatin gene activated. Reprinted from *Curr Opin Genet Dev*, 9, Lee S. J., McPherron A. C., 'Myostatin and the control of skeletal muscle mass', 604–7 (1999), with permission from Elsevier.

expression of different versions of modified myostatin in mice, resulting in increased muscle mass (Zhu *et al.*, 2000; Lee and McPherron, 2001; Yang et al., 2001). Also expression of other factors interfering with myostatin has been shown to increase muscle size, e.g. follistatin (Lee and McPherron, 2001).

VEGF

While none of the above mentioned genes yet have been tested on humans, similar effects as in mice and monkeys would be expected. One candidate for gene doping that has been tested on humans is the vascular endothelial growth factor (VEGF). VEGF is a growth factor for blood vessels and is among the front runners in gene therapy trials. Many elderly people have problems with the blood supply to the limbs due to a reduction in the number of blood vessels, in the worst cases causing ischemia in the extremities leading to amputations of the limbs. Since the patients simply need new blood vessels to replace the dead ones VEGF gene therapy is considered a promising solution. By using a virus carrying an activated VEGF gene and injecting this virus into the limbs of such patients, it has been demonstrated

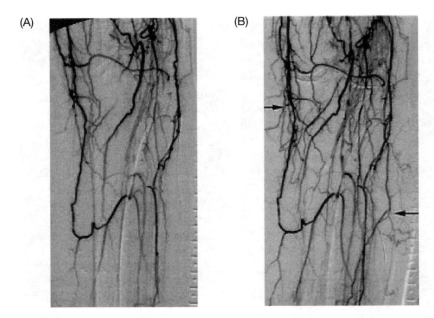

Figure 2.4 Increase in blood vessels by VEGF gene therapy in humans. Contrast picture of blood vessels in the leg of a patient before (A) and 8 weeks after (B) injection with an activated VEGF gene. Reprinted from Baumgartner I., Pieczek A., Manor O., Blair R., Kearney M., Walsh K., Isner J. M. (1998) 'Constitutive expression of phVEGF165 after intramuscular gene transfer promotes collateral vessel development in patients with critical limb ischemia', *Circulation*, 97: 1114–23, with permission from Lippincott Williams & Wilkins.

that new blood vessels are formed and the blood flow within the limbs improved (Baumgartner *et al.*, 1998) (Figure 2.4).

Increasing the blood flow in the muscles of endurance athletes might have a beneficial effect on their performance. Since the construct already exists for human use, although only in the laboratories, in principle, this already offers an opportunity for misuse today.

FUTURE POSSIBILITIES

When gene therapy becomes an established technique, then most likely artificial genes developed specifically for gene doping will emerge. Here there would be many possibilities to improve the human body.

Transcription factors

The examples given above of the possibilities today all concern the use of genes for hormones. The reason for this is that hormones function between cells and, therefore, modification in one cell can have an effect on many more cells. So even if the efficiency of introducing the artificial gene is low, a substantial effect can be achieved. However, the use of hormones also limits the possibilities of specific changes that can be achieved. A much broader span of possibilities opens up if genes for transcription factors are used. Transcription factors are the proteins within the cell that govern the activity of genes. So by expressing the correct transcription factor within a cell, many different genes can be activated or down-regulated. For instance, muscle fibres contain transcription factors which control the genes for oxidative enzymes, so by expressing these transcription factors in the muscle fibres, the oxidative profile can be improved (Ekmark *et al.*, 2003; Lin *et al.*, 2002). The current problem when using transcription factors is the efficiency of transferring the artificial gene into cells. Whereas a very small fraction of cells need to be genetically modified with hormone genes to accomplish a large effect, with transcription factors a substantial fraction of the cells need to be modified to achieve a significant effect since only the modified cells will change phenotype. However, the efficiencies of delivering the artificial genes are continuously improving, so the use of transcription factors most likely will become feasible.

Further in the future it might even be possible not only to optimize the existing phenotype, but to actually construct new phenotypes. In other tissues or other animals better protein versions may exist which could then be expressed in the relevant tissue. For instance, the human genome contains the gene for a contractile protein that is even faster than the ones expressed in normal muscles, and one could imagine that this 'silent' gene could be forced to be expressed in the normal muscles, giving rise to a superfast sprinter (Andersen *et al.*, 2000).

Fine-tuning the genetic make-up

Today it is only possible to add new genes but not to change the existing ones in the human body cells. However, in future it might be possible to change the existing genes (Kmiec, 2003). Together with the increasing knowledge about the small differences within genes that give rise to the genetic differences between the athletes, one can imagine that in future it might be possible to fine-tune the genetic make-up of an athlete to have the best versions of the relevant genes.

POTENTIAL HEALTH RISKS

Gene therapy is a new medical treatment with vast potentials. However, gene therapy experiments have been hit by a couple of very unfortunate accidents where patients have died from the treatment. The first major setback for gene therapy was in 1999 when 18-year-old Jesse Gelsinger died from a gene therapy treatment

(Hollon, 2000). He had a defect gene for an enzyme in the nitrogen metabolism, ornithine transcarboxylase, and was injected with a virus carrying a healthy copy of the gene. Apparently, his body responded so vigorously to the infection by the virus itself that he died from multiple organ failure. Recently, a gene therapy trial to cure severe immunodeficiency in children caused cancer in two of the children (Hacein-Bey-Abina et al., 2003). Although these accidents seem problematic, they appear to be special cases that can be avoided in other trials. However, the progress in gene therapy trials has been slowed down due to the very high security measures that have been imposed on such trials in order to prevent new unexpected deaths.

Too much EPO production

Since it is still difficult to control the activity of the new gene, the risk of over-production is very high. For instance, the overproduction of EPO will cause too high hematocrit levels which can lead to heart failure. However, in future this problem may be reduced due to the development of regulatory promoters. However, even if production can be controlled, it would still be necessary to monitor the production level, which would require the participation of doctors. So it might not be possible for the athletes to use these constructs on their own without the involvement of a physician. However, for many other gene doping targets, such as growth factors, overproduction might not be a serious problem and therefore EPO could be taken by the individual athlete alone.

Side effects

Most normal drugs have side effects to some degree, ranging from stomach pains and headaches to sudden death. The same will be expected from gene therapy, but the problem is more severe in this case. With normal drugs, in the case of serious side effects, the administration of the drug can be terminated. However, for gene therapy there is normally no way to stop the treatment if problems arise, which makes side effects a much bigger problem in gene therapy. As mentioned earlier, research is, however, underway to try to build in suicide genes that can be used to terminate the treatment in case of trouble.

Immune response

Since nowadays most gene therapy constructs include foreign protein from viruses or bacteria, the immune system may activate a response to this which can lead to elimination of the target cells or in the worst cases, a general immune overreaction causing multiple organ failure. The overreaction to the virus was probably what killed Jesse Gersinger and potentially it could also kill the experimenting athlete. For normal gene therapy use, this problem is anticipated and measures are taken to avoid it.

Autoimmunization

Recently, another surprising problem has emerged. In some cases the gene therapy can deceive the immune system into considering both the produced protein as well as the endogenous as foreign. When EPO gene therapy was tested on monkeys some of the monkeys developed an autoimmune response to EPO, causing a *fall* in hematocrit rather than the expected rise (Gao *et al.*, 2004; Chenuaud *et al.*, 2004). The reason for this is yet unknown, but could create a serious problem if this happens in an athlete trying to boost his or her normal production of EPO or other hormones.

Cancer

Since the DNA can get integrated into the genome, the risk of cancer is always present. Integration will alter the gene that the construct by chance happens to be integrated into. Cancer is due to unfortunate alterations of genes so the possibility of cancer cannot be ruled out. In fact, the two recent cases of cancer caused by gene therapy treatment of immunodeficiency were most likely due to integration into a latent cancer gene (Hacein-Bey-Abina *et al.*, 2003).

CONCLUSION

Currently, gene therapy is still a very dangerous technique and only the most foolish athlete would try to use it for doping at present. Furthermore, the treatments are only available in only a few experimental laboratories. However, as gene therapy becomes a more established technique and approved for normal treatments, the treatments will be much more easily available and safer to use. Even then, due to the huge power of gene therapy, the potential risks are still very high when used in uncontrolled environments. So if athletes start using it on their own, we will see some bad cases. On the other hand, due to the current high focus on safety, in a controlled environment it might be relatively safe in the future. Perhaps the danger would be relatively small if used in organized sports teams where physicians are involved as well. However, the physicians may also be pressed to allow the use to go too far to achieve the maximal effect.

REFERENCES

Agha-Mohammadi, S. and Lotze, M.T. (2000) 'Regulatable systems: applications in gene therapy and replicating viruses', *Journal of Clinical Investigations*, 105: 1177–83.

Andersen, J.L., Schjerling, P. and Saltin, B. (2002) 'Muscle, genes and athletic performance', *Scientific American*, 283: 48–55.

Ataka, K., Maruyama, H., Neichi, T., Miyazaki, J. and Gejyo, F. (2003) 'Effects of erythropoietin-gene electrotransfer in rats with adenine-induced renal failure'. *American Journal of Nephrology*, 23: 315–23.

Barton-Davis, E.R., Shoturma, D.I., Musaro, A., Rosenthal, N. and Sweeney, H.L. (1998) 'Viral mediated expression of insulin-like growth factor I blocks the aging-related loss of skeletal muscle function', *Proceedings of the National Academy of Science, USA*, 95: 15603–7.

Baumgartner, I., Pieczek, A., Manor, O., Blair, R., Kearney, M., Walsh, K. and Isner, J.M. (1998) Constitutive expression of phVEGF165 after intramuscular gene transfer promotes collateral vessel development in patients with critical limb ischemia', *Circulation*, 97: 1114–23.

Bohl, D., Salvetti, A., Moullier, P. and Heard, J.M. (1998) 'Control of erythropoietin delivery by doxycycline in mice after intramuscular injection of adeno-associated vector', *Blood*, 92: 1512–17.

Chenuaud, P., Larchet, T., Rabinowitz, J.E., Provost, N., Cherel, Y., Casadevall, N., Samulski, R.J. and Moullier, P. (2004) 'Autoimmune anemia in macaques following erythropoietin gene therapy', *Blood*, 103: 3303–4.

Ekmark, M., Gronevik, E., Schjerling, P. and Gundersen, K. (2003) 'Myogenin induces higher oxidative capacity in pre-existing mouse muscle fibres after somatic DNA transfer', *Journal of Physiology*, (2003) 548: 259–69.

Gao, G., Lebherz, C., Weiner, D.J., Grant, R., Calcedo, R., Bagg, A., Zhang, Y. and Wilson, J.M. (2004) 'Erythropoietin gene therapy leads to autoimmune anemia in macaques', *Blood*, 103: 3300–2.

Hacein-Bey-Abina, S., Von Kalle, C., Schmidt, M., McCormack, M.P., Wulffraat, N., Leboulch, P. *et al.* (2003) 'LMO2-associated clonal T cell proliferation in two patients after gene therapy for SCID-X1', *Science*, 302: 415–19.

Hollon, T. (2000) 'Researchers and regulators reflect on first gene therapy death', *Nature Medicine* 6: 6.

Hundevadt, K. (1998) 'Muskelsvindlerne', *Jyllands-Posten* 22 August.

Johnston, J., Tazelaar, J., Rivera, V.M., Clackson, T., Gao, G.P. and Wilson, J.M. (2003) 'Regulated expression of erythropoietin from an AAV vector safely improves the anemia of beta-thalassemia in a mouse model', *Molecular Therapy*, (2003) 7: 493–7.

Kmiec, E.B. (2003) 'Targeted gene repair – in the arena', *Journal of Clinical Investigation*, 112: 632–6.

Lee, S.J. and McPherron, A.C. (1999) 'Myostatin and the control of skeletal muscle mass', *Current Opinion in Genetics and Development*, (1999) 9: 604–7.

Lee, S.J. and McPherron, A.C. (2001) 'Regulation of myostatin activity and muscle growth', *Proceedings of the National Academy of Science*, 98: 9306–11.

Lin, J., Wu, H., Tarr, P.T., Zhang, C.Y., Wu, Z., Boss, O., Michael, L.F., Puigserver, P., Isotani, E., Olson, E.N., Lowell, B.B., Bassel-Duby, R. and Spiegelman, B.M. (2002) 'Transcriptional co-activator PGC-1 alpha drives the formation of slow-twitch muscle fibres', *Nature*, 418: 797–801.

McCrory, P. (2003) 'Super athletes or gene cheats?' *British Journal of Sports Medicine*, 37: 192–3.

McPherron, A.C., Lawler, A.M. and Lee, S.J. (1997) 'Regulation of skeletal muscle mass in mice by a new TGF-beta superfamily member', *Nature*, 387: 83–90.

Nordstrom, J.L. (2003) 'The antiprogestin-dependent GeneSwitch system for regulated gene therapy', *Steroids*, 68: 1085–94.

Rizzuto, G., Cappelletti, M., Maione, D., Savino, R., Lazzaro, D., Costa, P., Mathiesen, I., Cortese, R., Ciliberto, G., Laufer, R., La Monica, N. and Fattori, E. (1999) Efficient and regulated erythropoietin production by naked DNA injection and muscle electroporation', *Proceedings of the National Academy of Science, USA*, 96: 6417–22.

Siprashvili, Z. and Khavari, P.A. (2004) 'Lentivectors for regulated and reversible cutaneous gene delivery', *Molecular Therapy*, 9: 93–100.

Svensson, E.C., Black, H.B., Dugger, D.L., Tripathy, S.K., Goldwasser, E., Hao, Z., Chu, L. and Leiden, J.M. (1997) 'Long-term erythropoietin expression in rodents and non-human primates following intramuscular injection of a replication-defective adenoviral vector', *Human Gene Therapy*, 8: 1797–806.

Terada, Y., Tanaka, H., Okado, T., Shimamura, H., Inoshita, S., Kuwahara, M., Akiba, T. and Sasaki, S. (2002) 'Ligand-regulatable erythropoietin production by plasmid injection and in vivo electroporation', *Kidney International* 62: 1966–76.

Tripathy, S.K., Goldwasser, E., Lu, M.M., Barr, E. and Leiden, J.M. (1994) 'Stable delivery of physiologic levels of recombinant erythropoietin to the systemic circulation by intramuscular injection of replication-defective adenovirus', *Proceedings of the National Academy of Science, USA*, 91: 11557–61.

Yang, J., Ratovitski, T., Brady, J.P., Solomon, M.B., Wells, K.D. and Wall, R.J. (2001) 'Expression of myostatin pro domain results in muscular transgenic mice', *Molecular Reproduction and Development*, 60: 351–61.

Ye, X., Rivera, V.M., Zoltick, P., Cerasoli, F. Jr, Schnell, M.A., Gao, G., Hughes, J.V., Gilman, M. and Wilson, J.M. (1999) 'Regulated delivery of therapeutic proteins after in vivo somatic cell gene transfer', *Science*, 283: 88–91.

Zhou, S., Murphy, J.E., Escobedo, J.A. and Dwarki, V.J. (1998) 'Adeno-associated virus-mediated delivery of erythropoietin leads to sustained elevation of hematocrit in nonhuman primates', *Gene Therapy*, 5: 665–70.

Zhu, X., Hadhazy, M., Wehling, M., Tidball, J.G. and McNally, E.M. (2000) 'Dominant negative myostatin produces hypertrophy without hyperplasia in muscle', *Federation of European Biochemical Societies Letters*, 474: 71–5.

3 Genetic enhancement of athletic performance

Angela J. Schneider

Gene transfer technology offers enormous promise. It is expected that gene transfer technology will revolutionize the way we view illness and health and that gene transfer technology will transform the way we treat and prevent disease. If the social impact of gene transfer technology is likely to be unprecedented, its effect on sport will be just as momentous. Some of the predictions for the effect of the genetic revolution have been grave. The human genome has been called the book of life, the repository of all that is human. Deciphering that book of life is taken to offer the key to wonderful new genetic treatments and technologies that can transform the way we think of illness and treatment, and the normal limits of life itself. Going further, understanding – and then being able to manipulate – human genetics offers the prospect of specifically designing human beings to have particular aptitudes and characteristics. But because all current work on gene transfer technology is in the research stage, its potential impact is as yet unknown. The imminent applications to sport performance include muscle growth factors and oxygen transport and utilization. The World Anti-Doping Agency was well aware of these potential applications to sport when it hosted the Banbury Workshop on Genetic Enhancement of Athletic Performance at the Banbury Center, Cold Spring Harbour Laboratory, New York from 17–20 March 2002. This workshop brought together international experts and leaders in biology and genetics, sports medicine, ethicists, policy-makers, legal experts, representatives of the Olympic Movement and athletes to explore the science, technology, and ethical issues facing the sports community as a consequence of gene transfer technology.

During the process of the two-and-one-half day workshop on Genetic Enhancement of Athletic Performance, it was agreed that a combination of regulation, education, and research is the best current method for addressing the prospect of gene doping in sport from becoming a reality. WADA Chairman, Richard W. Pound, stated, 'Gene therapy has enormous potential to revolutionize medicine's approach to curing disease and improving the quality of life. Unfortunately, this same technology, like many others, can be abused to enhance athletic performance,' and that

> WADA is committed to confronting the possible misuse of gene transfer technology in sport. The same kinds of people who cheat in sport today will

probably try to find ways to misuse genetics tomorrow. WADA is grateful to all those who helped us gain an understanding of this new field so we can consider how best to respond to the possible misuses.[1]

Further, Mr Pound concluded that,

> We found a remarkable degree of confluence amongst the scientific and sport representatives regarding the possibilities of benefit to the community at large from developments in genetic therapy, the need for a properly considered social framework for such activities, and the need to prevent the misuse of this developing branch of science.[2]

Dr Ted Friedmann, Professor of Pediatrics at the University of California San Diego, Center for Molecular Genetics, claimed that, 'We must underscore that the work on genetic therapies should be considered research, promising for the future betterment of mankind but still unpredictable and of unproven safety.'[3] Dr Friedmann concluded that, 'The time is right, however, for the sport and science communities to begin working out how to prevent the possible misuse of these methods in the future.'[4]

The Banbury Conference was truly a unique and 'cutting edge' gathering of specialists and experts attending with the express intention of exploring current developments in gene transfer technology and their potential impact on sport. This conference was important for WADA because part of its mission is to foster a doping-free culture in sport.[5] It combines the resources of sport and government to enhance, supplement and coordinate existing efforts to educate athletes about the harms of doping, to reinforce the ideal of fair play and to sanction those who cheat themselves and their sport.[6]

The Banbury Workshop participants came to a series of conclusions, some general and other specific to sport.[7] The more general conclusions were as follows:

1   Gene transfer technology, which is still at the investigational stage, is nevertheless already beginning to demonstrate clinical efficacy.
2   While genetic technologies hold immense therapeutic promise, there is potential for their misuse, including attempts at the enhancement of athletic performance.
3   The collective efforts of scientists, ethicists, athletes, sports authorities, medical practitioners, professional societies, pharmaceutical and biotech industries, and public authorities (including governments) will be required to avert such misuse.
4   The compliance with established international standards pertaining to genetic experimentation involving human subjects, such as the Helsinki, Geneva, and Inuyama Declarations that prevent unethical research is essential. (The application of genetic transfer technologies should be consistent with established standards of professional behaviour.)

5   The pace of research in the field of genetic transfer technology is such that governmental and other regulatory agencies must work with a continued sense of urgency to establish a social and policy framework to guide this research and its applications and sanction breaches of the framework.

6   Broad public discussion and the development of social and policy frameworks must surround the distinction between genetic therapy and genetic enhancement. The time for the social framework to be established is before abuses occur, not after-the-fact.

The sport specific conclusions were as follows:

1   Athletes, in common with other people in society, are entitled to the benefits of genuine therapeutic applications to treat injuries and other medical conditions.

2   There are evident risks that genetic transfer technologies might be used in a manner that would be contrary to the spirit of sport or potentially dangerous to the health of athletes. Akin to doping in the present generation, genetic transfer technology that is non-therapeutic and merely performance-enhancing should be prohibited.

3   The definition of doping used by WADA, the IOC, international sports federations (IFs), and national authorities should be expanded to include the unapproved use of genetic transfer technologies.

4   One of the benefits of genetic technology is its potential use in the detection of prohibited substances and methods.

5   The scientific community has recognized the need for the continued development and refinement of methods that will permit the detection of the misuse of genetic transfer technologies in sport. The workshop members noted there are a number of approaches that currently exist, or are in development, that will permit such detection.

6   The present focus of WADA's research grants toward the study of the detection methods for the misuse of oxygen-carrying agents and growth factors should be extended to include the detection of genetic transfer technologies and their effects.

7   The World Anti-Doping Code, which is planned for implementation by 2004, should include language prohibiting the use of genetic transfer technologies to enhance athletic performance.

8   WADA calls upon its government members, in particular, to expedite the development of a global social framework for the application of genetic transfer technologies that address the potential misuse of these technologies in sport and a publicly stated deadline for the adoption of that framework.

9   WADA calls upon governments to consider the following recommendations for inclusion in the regulatory framework pertaining to genetic transfer technologies and related research:

    (a) Address breaches of the social framework within the criminal or penal realm.

    (b) Extend corporate liability to directors, officers and senior employees.

(c) Extend civil and criminal limitation periods in respect of breaches of the regulatory framework.
(d) Require detailed record-keeping in respect of all applications of gene transfer technologies with independent audit requirements.
(e) Expand standards of medical and professional behaviour to prohibit the improper use of genetic transfer technologies and that such rules be actively enforced.

10 WADA calls upon governments and the sports movement to establish and fund educational and ethics programs designed to prevent the possible misuses of genetic transfer technologies in sport. WADA is willing to coordinate the design and dissemination of such programs.
11 WADA and the scientific community will establish a mechanism for continuing dialogue and consultation around the subject of genetic transfer technologies.

Given the conclusions of the Banbury workshop, there are a number of practical issues that arise and are important to identify. The first set is with regard to the current state of research. All inquiries into gene transfer technology are currently at the research phase. The procedures and techniques are not firmly fixed, nor are they commercially available. The research is currently subject to a range of regulatory and review procedures. Research on the human applications of gene transfer technology is highly regulated and reviewed at local and national levels in North America and to some extent, by similar mechanisms in other nations; however, review and regulation vary by jurisdiction and nation. From the sport perspective there are gaps in that regulation – in that, a study would not be likely to be described as having the purpose of exploring the enhancement of sport performance, though it could have that effect.[8] This situation presents both a challenge and an opportunity. The challenge is that in the absence of currently available protocols WADA has been asked to respond to hypothetical and perhaps highly fanciful possibilities.[9] The fact is that governments, sport organizations and WADA have the potential to influence development of regulation and review procedures at a very early stage.

A second set of practical issues arises around the possibility of testing. There was general agreement in the Banbury workshop that improved and more efficient methods are required to detect and test for genetic modification or the physiological effects of genetic modification.[10] Testing may well be difficult but it involves technical issues that are thought to be solvable by improved research and technology development. Methods for detection and testing could be aimed at both the primary genetic modification and secondary indicators.

One of these methods could involve the use of 'markers'. The principal (and principled) difficulty is that current genetic modifications are, in practical terms, untestable. However, there exists the possibility that genetic markers, for which there could be tests, could accompany modifications. The addition, though, of scientifically unnecessary markers raises serious ethical and scientific problems.

The ethical problem is that an unnecessary marker carries with it additional risks of harm. Because these risks are unnecessary from the perspective of research, and only necessary for the purpose of detecting doping in sport, they pose an unacceptable risk to research participants. In scientific terms, the addition of unnecessary markers provides an additional risk of compromising the research with the addition of potentially confounding variables. The incorporation of markers or tags into foreign therapeutic genes to make them more readily detectable may help in detection programs but would be contrary to best principles of drug design in which only therapeutic efficacy should be relevant.

Other than some serious practical issues, there are also some serious conceptual issues that need to be addressed.[11] The first conceptual issue involves drawing the line between therapy and enhancement. The standard approach in sport has been that 'therapy', a repair to bring one back to 'normal', has been permitted but 'enhancement' (going beyond 'normal') has been banned.[12] This approach does not fit neatly with current medical practice and thinking. For example, in many forms of prevention the body's normal responses to disease are enhanced to enable the person to avoid infection or illness. Second, a 'therapy' to repair muscle torn while engaged in strenuous weight training, would be a reaction to an injury caused by sport training and would, by enabling athletes to train harder and longer, enhance performance. Some muscle-repair 'therapies' would have the effect of making the muscle stronger than it was before the injury, thus enhancing performance. This issue is also at stake in endurance sports. Some sport physicians argue that the treatment provided to long-distance cyclists should be viewed as therapy to enable them to recover from their exertions. Others argue that the same interventions should be viewed as performance enhancing because they allow quicker recovery, enabling the athlete to compete again the next day. With gene transfer technology this issue will come to the fore. For example, treatments designed to enhance muscle repair and re-growth could well have the effect of enabling the muscle to grow stronger than it was before. Should such treatments be considered enhancements, and therefore banned?

The second conceptual issue that arises is related to harm.[13] At present, because gene transfer technology is still in the experimental stage, it is extremely risky and carries the potential of harm. One potential route would be to discourage, or ban, athlete participation in gene transfer technology research on the grounds that it is potentially both harmful and performance-enhancing. It could be argued that such a ban would be paternalistic and further it would be difficult to enforce, but the process of discouragement itself may be worth it if it could act as an educational tool that would get athletes thinking about some of the underlying issues and principles at stake.

The third conceptual issue arises around the relationship of sport to society. The way in which the public will treat gene transfer technology if and when it becomes readily available is unknown. For example, if muscle repair and re-growth technology develops sufficiently that older men are able to stem the tide of muscle loss through the use of gene transfer technology, then it is probably the case that such treatments will rapidly become available and widely used. If such treatments or enhancements became readily available and widely used, then it would be extremely difficult for sport to stand apart in opposition because sport operates in a social context. This, of course, is highly speculative. The practical implication of these possibilities is that governments, sport organizations and WADA need to monitor the development of the technology and public responses. It is probably prudent to adopt a flexible response that defends the spirit of sport but that leaves open the exact implications of that requirement in specific cases of gene transfer technology.

Despite the wide range of topics discussed at the Banbury workshop, there remain a number of critical issues that were not discussed. In sport it is anticipated that athletes will experiment with genetic treatments to aid recovery and then move quickly to enhancements of muscle mass and endurance. But, one of the worst-case scenarios is the prospect of designer athletes, a special breed of being, crafted specifically to excel at sport. Some of these issues perhaps remain within the realm of science fiction, but it behoves us to be thinking of possible responses in advance. There are ways in which we can reflect on the scientific advances within the context of sport and sport ethics. We can start with fundamental conceptions of sport ethics that drive the entire enterprise of doping and doping control in the first place. Unless we are sure and clear about just why it is that doping is such a bad thing that we should devote all this effort to eradicating it, we will be unable to face the challenges presented by new techniques of genetic doping. If we are agreed that it is important to avoid unnecessary risks of harm in sport, we can also use a variety of other – more problematic concepts and distinctions. Each of these distinctions is used in discussions of doping but the meaning of none of them is clear or uncontested. The reason for this is that the distinctions appear to be rooted in science (and hence are supposedly 'objective') when the truth is that these are conceptual distinctions that we, in this case, we the sport community, use for a variety of purposes.

In order to formulate an ethical response to the challenges of new genetic technologies we need to distinguish between different types of practice and different forms of treatment and enhancement. We can use two broad conceptual distinctions. The first is between the design of a new human being and the modification of a person who already exists. The second distinction, as outline above, is between a treatment and an enhancement. It should be noted that the distinctions between designing a new human, and modifying an existing person, and between treating a defect or injury and enhancing 'normal' functioning may be intuitively simple and compelling, but they do not map neatly onto different techniques in the science of genetics and it remains to be seen whether the distinctions are robust enough to withstand the philosophical challenges both face.

The first distinction involves 'genetic design'. This topic is probably far into the future, but it is one of the issues that is constantly raised in the media. Genetic design refers to the specific design of babies to have certain genetic traits or characteristics. As soon as this topic is raised, thoughts turn to the design of babies for sport performance. We should be unequivocal that such a prospect is fundamentally contrary to the spirit of sport, precisely because it views humans as the sorts of things that could be designed for sport, rather than recognizing that sport is a human creation, designed for our enjoyment.

The first distinction also involves 'germ-line therapy'. Germ-line therapy, versus the somatic gene transfer technology discussed above, also has practical and scientific issues concerning research into and application of the relevant technologies. Germ-line or heritable therapies were not discussed at the Banbury workshop. This category is not really about sport. The technologies to avoid genetic defects would not specifically create people for sport; their effect would merely be to increase the potential pool of healthy people able to participate in sport. Of course, there are broader social questions about whether we should use those technologies at all, and there are important issues about the implication of the use of such technologies would have for people who have the genetic diseases concerned or those who do not have access to the technology. But about these issues sport has nothing special to say. The puzzle posed concerning germ-line therapies would be the response to second-generation inheritors of genetic modifications passed through the germ line. These would be people who had won the genetic lottery – but had won because their parents had rigged the outcome. This development would put an organization like WADA in an impossible position. On the one hand, organizations like WADA would probably be opposed to the design of people for sport, on the other, these individuals would be innocent, it would have been their parents who did the designing (perhaps not specifically for sport) and the manipulated nature of their genetic inheritance may well be impossible to identify. At this stage the best response is probably one that relegates this possibility to the realm of science fiction and which reiterates opposition to the very idea of designing people for sport.

There are other uses of genetic technology, for example, genetic screening *in vitro*, or *in utero*. It is in principle possible to screen embryos for genetic characteristics and then either only implant into the womb, or carry to term, those with the 'desirable' genetic make-up. It is potentially possible to do this for genes associated with traits that predispose to greater athletic performance. The fate of athletes who had been born as a result of such a procedure was not discussed at the Banbury workshop, which focused on gene transfer technology. Again, such a possibility poses potentially serious concerns for an agency like WADA. On the one hand, such individuals would not have benefited from any artificial intervention with their genetic make-up. On the other hand, their genetic make-up would have been selected in order to maximize the chances of athletic success. Such individuals would be undetectable. Again, the best response may well be to reiterate opposition to designing people for sport while recognizing that, in practical terms, there is nothing an organization like WADA can do to detect or stop it. Another example concerns genetic screening *in vivo*. Genetic screening techniques could be used (as a form of potential aptitude testing) to determine which children or young people were most likely to be able to benefit from specialized sport training. Other than the novelty of this technique and other than issues of privacy (see below), the testing of young children for their sporting aptitude is a currently accepted practice, and one that need not involve an agency like WADA.

From the athlete's rights and human rights perspective, there are also important ethical issues those agencies like WADA must guard carefully against violating, for example – rights to privacy. In many respects athletes, as a population, present unique features as potential research subjects. Athletes are highly motivated; they are likely to be willing to sign up for even risky experimental treatments or therapies. They are also very likely to stick with the program until the end – athletes don't quit. Athletes are used to being in relationships where their physical actions and their food and nutrition are controlled by authority figures. Athletes build relationships with coaches, physiotherapists, sport psychologists, and so on, which accustom them to being told what to do with and about their bodies. Athletes are generally fit and healthy. This makes them an interesting and significant research population for it makes it possible to study the effect of an intervention on an otherwise healthy person. Athletes are therefore very appealing research subjects.

While the sport community has an important role to play in expressing its unequivocal opposition to the use of genetic therapies for enhancement purposes, the research community must also adopt a leadership position and show its commitment to not using athletes as research subjects where there is a reasonable expectation that the therapy under investigation will have a performance-enhancing effect. Genetic technology and the human genome raise a host of issues concerning individual privacy. Genetic information gathered for one purpose, perhaps therapy or treatment of a disease, may have significant repercussions in other areas of a person's life, e.g. eligibility for insurance. Some ethicists are currently advising that because no protection against discrimination (for instance, for eligibility for life insurance) exists for people who have a genetic predisposition to a disease, prudent people would decline from agreeing to any research, which identifies their genetic make-up. If agencies like WADA are going to be involved with any form of genetic testing, it will have to first satisfy those privacy concerns. If the human genome is the 'Book of Life', then my genetic make-up is the book of my life. Access to genetic information about individuals is access to information that is about as private as it can be. There remain great social questions about maintaining the privacy of personal genetic information. Sport needs to exercise caution that it does not become a wedge used to drive greater general access to genetic information.

In conclusion, there are also some things that sport can say about its own domain and the realm of genetic intervention to design people for sport. The IOC in its third Fundamental Principle, declares that: 'The goal of Olympism is to place everywhere sport at the service of the harmonious development of man, with a view to encouraging the establishment of a peaceful society concerned with the preservation of human dignity.'[14] Elsewhere in the Charter the IOC speaks of putting 'sport at the service of humanity' (Charter 2.2). The guardians of sport therefore have an obligation to ensure that their voices are heard loudly, clearly, and unequivocally condemning the possible use of genetic interventions to design humans for sport. Sport is just not that important – and it is up to those in sport to say so. Sport can, and should, be on record as saying that genetic design for the purposes of sport enhancement is totally antithetical to our conception of sport and its relationship to human lives. Sport is designed for people – people are not designed for sport!

PUBLIC CONSENT

The topic of 'public consent' is emerging as a trend in the examination of significant social ethical issues. Personal consent, as a requirement for treatment or experimentation, is a well-established principle. The aim of the doctrine of consent is to safeguard personal autonomy, the idea being that each person should, to the greatest extent possible, be able to make the important decisions that affect his or her life. The doctrine of consent requires that a person should be entitled to decide whether or not to undergo proposed treatments, therapies or experimental interventions. The doctrine of 'informed' consent adds the explanation that one cannot really give consent unless one knows what one is consenting to, in particular, unless one can assess the risks and benefits.

The notion of 'public consent' has developed because it is recognized that the doctrine of personal consent does not sufficiently safeguard those who are not themselves undergoing the treatment or therapy, yet who might be adversely affected.

The concept of public consent has broad applicability, but is especially useful if we consider it in the sport context. Sport forms a community with its own internal rules and regulations and standards of behaviour. Each sport is itself a rule-governed activity and members of the sporting community are entitled to expect that participants play by the rules. Where that expectation is not met, sport has the right – indeed the obligation – to defend its standards and values.

Personal consent to a treatment or practice, or to a research intervention, does not trump, or defeat sport's right to give or withhold its public consent. Individuals, through the exercise of their personal freedoms, are not entitled to undermine the entire practice of sport as a public good. And this applies to individual athletes, individual medical practitioners and individual researchers. While the formal mechanisms for seeking – and giving or withholding – public consent are not yet in place (the nearest we get is the political process), WADA is in a unique position to focus this question for sport. WADA brings together both sport organizations and public authorities in an attempt to defend our vision of sport against those who threaten it by doping. This is the nearest thing we have to a process for giving or withholding public consent to genetic doping.

NOTES

1 'WADA conference sheds light on the potential of gene doping.' WADA media report, 20 March 2002, p. 1.
2 Ibid. p. 1.
3 Ibid. p. 1.

4 Ibid. p. 1.
5 www.wada-ama.org.
6 Ibid.
7 These conclusions were all outlined in the WADA media report cited above.
8 This issue and the others that follow were identified by A. Schneider at the Banbury Workshop.
9 This began at the media conference which immediately followed the Banbury Workshop.
10 This was noted in the media report and at the media conference that followed.
11 The conceptual issues were also identified by A. Schneider at the workshop.
12 This kind of language has been commonly used in the philosophy of sport literature on doping.
13 This issue is similar to that addressed in the doping in sport literature. I have dealt with this topic extensively in earlier publications (see Further Reading) so I will not repeat those arguments here.
14 Fundamental Principles #3 in Olympic Charter.

FURTHER READING

Schneider, A.J. (1993) 'Doping in Sport and the Perversion Argument', in G. Gaebauer (ed.) *The Relevance of the Philosophy of Sport.* (Berlin: Academia Verlag), pp. 117–28.

Schneider, A.J. with R.B. Butcher (1994) 'Why Olympic Athletes Should Avoid the Use and Seek the Elimination of Performance-Enhancing Substances and Practices in the Olympic Games', *Journal of the Philosophy of Sport*, Vols. XX and XXI: 64–81.

Schneider, A.J. and Butcher, R.B. (2000a) 'A Philosophical Overview of the Arguments on Banning Doping in Sport', in C.M. Tamburrini and T. Tännsjö (eds), *Values in Sport: Elitism, Nationalism, Gender Equality and the Scientific Manufacture of Winners* (London: E & FN Spon), pp. 185–200.

Schneider, A.J. and Butcher, R.B. (2000b) 'An Ethical Analysis of Drug Testing', in W. Wilson and E.A. Derse (eds) *Doping in Elite Sport: The Politics of Drugs in the Olympic Movement.* (Champaign, IL: Human Kinetics, 2000), pp. 102–24.

4 Gene doping

The shape of things to come

Andy Miah

INTRODUCTION

In recent years, the use of gene transfer technology in sport has become a critical issue for anti-doping authorities and sport ethicists.[1] Moreover, the subject continues to be the source of press coverage on the state of elite sport.[2] Over the past few years, these discussions have been translated into policy decisions about genetic technology from the perspectives of the International Olympic Committee (IOC) and the World Anti-Doping Agency (WADA). In 2001, the IOC developed a working group on gene therapy in sport and in 2002, WADA hosted a meeting to discuss the matter. In 2003, WADA included a reference to gene doping in their draft 2004 Anti-Doping Code, which makes the following prohibition:

II. PROHIBITED METHODS . . .

C. GENE DOPING

Gene or cell doping is defined as the non-therapeutic use of genes, genetic elements and/or cells that have the capacity to enhance athletic performance
(WADA, 2003)

A number of issues arise from this new policy on the parameters of acceptable performances in sport. For instance, no longer can it be argued that genetic modification might yet be legal, just because the rules did not prohibit the technology. Also, one might question why it is that this issue has gained such attention in the past few years, when genetic science has advanced relatively slowly. Moreover, one can ask whether making of policy on this matter is solely the concern of sporting authorities.

The focus of this chapter will be to question precisely these matters. I will inquire into the state of discussions on gene doping and recommend directions based on what immediate priorities exist in this area. Moreover, I will argue that the way in which this issue is being constructed in various contexts demonstrates why this innovation in sport performance cannot be treated in the same way as other enhancement methods. It is on this basis that I will doubt the substantive concerns about genetically modified athletes from the perspective of sporting organisations and why I will advocate a more central role for broader bioethical discussions on policy related to gene doping.

WHY WORRY ABOUT GENETICALLY MODIFIED ATHLETES?

Many experts contest the value of discussing the prospect of genetically modified athletes. Indeed, Steve Jones commented at the Genes in Sport conference at University College London in 2001 that, 'there is a massive quantity of hype when it comes to gene therapy in sport. I put it in the same ballpark as the babbling nonsense talked about a baldness cure based on gene therapy' (cited in Powell, 2001). One might imagine that this is reason enough to reflect on the importance of discussing this matter, though the entire history and value of genetic science are contested for similar kinds of reasons. The progress made in genetic science in the past twenty years has been slow and the application of therapeutic interventions remains limited. As such, the prospect of utilising such technology to enhance a human being (an athlete) is often dismissed as obviously unethical, just because this technology is clearly not at all safe or possible yet.[3] On this basis, WADA might as well include in their anti-doping policy a prohibition of using 'the Force' for any potential athlete-Jedi wannabes. (Just for clarification, 'the Force' is not yet prohibited by WADA.) Yet, clearly some people consider the science sufficiently feasible, such that athletes might endeavour to capitalise on an imperfect scientific basis, if it means it might boost their performance.

I do not mean to appear dismissive of WADA's attempt to remain 'ahead' of the athletes, which is often given as a reason for why this topic is of interest to sporting officials at this particular time. Yet, I am not convinced that being ahead of the 'cheaters' is best approached by re-writing anti-doping policy and would like to think more carefully about what it would mean for anti-doping authorities to be 'ahead' of the athletes. Such an approach seems only to reinforce the power differential of athletes and the doping police.

As yet, there has been little sustained ethical discussion on gene doping. If one were to compare it with something like genetically modified food or crops, or even cloning, then it would not seem to have raised such a broad range of social concerns. Indeed, it would also appear that maintaining what is ethical about sport in the context of gene doping means trying to ensure that the use of this technology by athletes is effectively prohibited, rather than questioning whether genetically modified athletes are unethical at all. I am aware that, for many, ensuring doping does not take place in sport is one of its core ethical priorities. On such a view, doping compromises what is ethically valuable about sports. The difficult part for sports ethicists has been trying to establish precisely what it is that doping compromises, though I shall not go too far into this matter here. It is discussed widely in other articles on doping and elsewhere in this volume in relation to gene doping.

Instead, I wish to explore how this topic has become part of the doping agenda and to do so by examining quite different examples of how this issue has been discussed. Together, these examples reveal how the subject of gene doping might be approached from very different perspectives, which demonstrate various ways of thinking about the ethics of this technology. However, first, some clarification about the kind of research that has taken place, which suggests why gene doping is something to think about very seriously, will be useful.

THE SCIENCE OF GENE DOPING

Genetic science is not at a point where it is possible to genetically enhance athletes safely, nor is such technology likely to be medically safe for some years, if, indeed, it ever will be. Also, it is important to recognise that the kinds of modifications that might appear in the near future will not be the very specific applications that are sometimes imagined in futuristic scenarios portrayed in newspaper tabloids and magazines. Thus, we will have no gene for a javelin-thrower's arm or a gene that can allow an athlete to perform a quadruple axel in skating. Instead, we might discover effective ways of harnessing genes related to endurance or strength, which will be useful for a range of human pursuits, of which sport might be one.

It is possible to identify a number of emerging studies in genetic science, which could lead to such applications in sport (Pérusse et al., 2003). For example, IGF-1 or insulin-like growth factor might be used by athletes to boost muscle mass, even though its medical purpose is for treating a muscle-wasting disease (Barton-Davis et al., 1998; Goldspink, 2001). Using a form of IGF-1 called mechano growth factor (MGF) with mice, which is used to treat muscle-wasting diseases such as muscular dystrophy, Goldspink's team were able to isolate muscle tissue and insert the MGF gene. The results show an increase in muscle mass by approximately 20 per cent after two weeks. At Harvard University, Dr Nadia Rosenthal used IGF-1 in gene therapy in mice to halt depletion of muscle strength that comes with old age. As Rosenthal notes:

> Older mice increased their muscle strength by as much as 27 percent in the experiment, which suggested possibilities for athletes as well as for preserving muscle strength in elderly people and increasing muscle power in those who suffer from muscular dystrophy.
>
> (cited in Longman, 2001, html)

Additionally, genetically engineered erythropoietin (EPO) might be used to boost an athlete's performance on the genetic level. EPO has the potential to increase endurance capabilities, though its medical application is to increase the hematocrit level in patients with chronic renal disease. Research identifies the effects of inserting genes into a virus to produce a specific bodily effect, such as for the case of Svensson et al. (1997), which utilises an adenovirus to deliver EPO to mice and monkeys to observe whether it would render a difference in biological capabilities. By inserting the gene into a virus strand, it was transported throughout the body and did, indeed, have the effect of increasing the level of red blood cells that were being pumped around the body. In performance, this produces a similar effect to that of blood-doping, which operates on a similar principle by re-introducing blood into the body to boost the amount of oxygen being transported around the body, to offset fatigue. Thus, genetically inserting EPO into an athlete could increase the capabilities for endurance when active, which would be useful for any long-distance event.

Other emerging research from Lin *et al.* (2002) includes the gene 'PGC-1∞', which is known to tell other genes in the muscle whether they should be turned on or off. The implications of manipulating this gene entail the possibility of being able to switch on those muscle fibres (fast or slow twitch) that are most conducive to an athlete's chosen sport. Alternatively, variations in the ACE gene (angiotensin-converting enzyme) have been associated with endurance capabilities and an anabolic response to intense exercise training (Gayagay *et al.* 1998; Montgomery *et al.* 1998, 1999; Taylor *et al.* 1999; Brull *et al.* 2001; Plata *et al.* 2002). Williams, *et al.* (2000) studied this enzyme by comparing two groups of athletes, one with a strong ACE presence and one with low ACE presence. As Anderson (2000: html) explains:

> The angiotensin-converting-enzyme story begins with a plasma protein called angiotensinogen, which is present in the blood of all human beings. Under certain conditions, kidney cells secrete a hormone called renin into the blood which cleaves a 10-amino-acid protein from angiotensinogen to form a compound called angiotensin I. The various physiological roles played by angiotensin I are not completely understood, but it is known that angiotensin-converting enzyme (ACE) can knock two amino acids off angiotensin I to form a compound called angiotensin II. Angiotensin II has a variety of functions, but for purposes of our discussion we can simply say that it directly increases blood pressure by constricting arteries, and it indirectly raises blood pressure and blood volume by stimulating thirst centres in the brain and directing the kidneys to conserve more minerals and water.

ALTERNATIVE VIEWS ON GENE DOPING

The World Anti-Doping Agency and the International Olympic Committee have not been alone in taking an interest in how genetic technology might be used for sport. On 11 July 2002, the United States President's Council on Bioethics met to discuss the prospect of genetic manipulation for sport (US President's Council on Bioethics, 2002). The Council received a presentation from Dr Theodore Friedmann (UCLA), who also serves on the WADA Health and Medical Research Committee, and who has been involved with this topic for some time. Dr Friedmann outlined the scientific possibilities and together with the Council, discussed the ethical implications of the technology. Additionally, the Australian Law Reforms Commission (ALRC, 2003) has demonstrated a concern about the use of genetic information for sport. We shall now discuss both these institutions' views on gene doping.

The US President's Council on Bioethics

The President's Council meeting presents a quite different kind of discourse to the IOC and WADA meetings.[4] Consulting the minutes of the meeting, one has the impression that the Council is less concerned with sporting values and protecting the alleged integrity of sport. It is not that this 'integrity' is overlooked, but that the perspectives emerging from the meeting are varied. They can be summarised as follows:

- the Romantic View
- the Entertainment View
- the Techno-Centred View.

The 'Romantic View' is most comparable to that asserted by the IOC and WADA and is concerned with the alleged integrity of sport, which is seen as being threatened by the genetic technology. The 'Entertainment View' recognises sport as an entertaining enterprise, where it is valued primarily for providing extraordinary performances. In this case, genetic modification could enhance the entertainment value of sport and thus would be desirable. Finally, the 'Techno-Centred View' of sport considers sports to be constitutively technology. Consequently, genetic modification in sport is the sophistication of sport's inherently technological character and can be legitimate for this reason.

The Council also raises some general points of argumentation, contrasting 'individual autonomy' perspectives with 'social practice' concerns. Here, the Council engages with the ethical limits of paternalism, recognising that, if athletes are fully informed of the risks, then there seems no reason to prevent them from using such technology. However, it was also recognised that since genetic technology is at such an early stage, it is not currently possible for athletes to claim that they are 'informed' since we simply do not know enough about the risks. In this sense, autonomy might be compromised since, without knowing the risks, one cannot be informed enough to make a decision.[5] It was also recognised that the genetic issue in sport is comparable to the performance modification questions in sports more generally. The Council also questions the role of medicine in the process towards permitting the use of gene transfer technology in sport. Of interest has been the problematisation of the therapy/enhancement distinction and the epistemological difficulties of asserting what constitutes a 'normal' disposition, from which one can reject being 'abnormal'.

In sum, the President's Council arguments appear to prioritise concerns about safety, fairness, and character, where character is their primary moral concern. Both safety and fairness are secondary issues, since each could be overcome while maintaining the moral integrity of sport. Certainly, Council members were not convinced that genetic modification might make sport fairer, though this is not only because we cannot know the outcome of genetic modification and whether it might affect different people in different ways. Rather, and more persuasively, their contention is that it cannot be concluded that one individual is genetically superior than another. For example, let us suppose that the phenotypes of two endurance athletes could be compared and it were possible to identify the capability of their respective 'endurance genes'. In making its claim, the Council argues that a difference between the athletes does not permit the conclusion that one athlete is genetically superior to the other, since that would be to prioritise the value of only one gene rather than giving a balanced appraisal of the genetic capabilities of each individual. For this reason, genetic superiority cannot be used as a basis for concluding that genetic modification is legitimate to equalise athletes.

In conclusion, the Council concluded that what matters most in sport are the 'means' by which achievements are gained and that this is largely related to appraising the character of the athlete. On this basis, genetic modification has little value because it does not have any bearing on the athlete's character and to allow its use would make it more difficult to appraise the capabilities of the athlete.

The Australian Law Reforms Council

The ALRC has an approach comparable to the US President's Council. It appears to have neither a preconceived notion of sporting values, nor any strong appreciation for sport ethics, or even ethics *per se*.[6] Rather, its concern is for the legal implications of using genetic information. Their perspective is interesting for sports ethicists largely because it is quite distinct from the other discussions, which focus on emerging and, for some, futuristic technology. In contrast, the ALRC concerns rely upon comparably rudimentary technology, though which still give rise to considerable ethical and legal concerns. Their discussion paper about the use of genetic information agrees that sporting authorities might misuse such information to the detriment of individual athletes' rights. For example, the ALRC state that:

> genetic testing may lead to discrimination against certain athletes. For example, an athlete with a susceptibility to a particular injury may never in fact develop the injury, but may be dropped from the team by management in an effort to avoid potential liability if the injury manifests. Alternatively, a sports co-ordination body may seek to impose certain conditions on players to minimise its own liability for any injuries they may suffer. For example, the Professional Boxing and Martial Arts Board (Vic) has proposed the genetic testing of all professional boxers in Victoria as a condition of their license to fight.
>
> (ALRC, 2003)

The ALRC approach is also more critical than the IOC, WADA, or even the US President's Council. What is most noticeable about their approach is the concern for how a genetically modified human might be affected by policy in sport. They recognise that the existence of genetically modified persons – athletes or otherwise – cannot simply entail the disqualification of such persons from social practices.

Interestingly, this specific matter of how genetic information might be used (in contrast to genetic modification) has not attracted the attention of other official organisations. Indeed, IOC President Jacques Rogge noted in 2001 that he saw no reason why genetic information might not be used to discover which sports people are best suited to (Rogge, cited in Clarey, 2001). Jacques Rogge, a medical surgeon and former Olympian, will perhaps not have intended his statement to legitimize the search for 'performance genes', when such possibilities seem only partial at best presently. Nevertheless, even making this admission, the correlation of phenotypes with athletic performance is ethically complex. Subjecting athletes (including children) to genetic tests in order to determine whether they have been enhanced also involves a number of ethical issues, which do not seem to have attracted much attention. This is surprising since the ethical issues arising from the use and abuse of genetic information seem the most immediate, given that they do not rely significantly on future technology.

The implications of these discussions are rather unclear, since neither the ALRC nor the US President's Council has any clear mandate for deciding what is ethical in sport. Yet, the ramifications of the ALRC conclusions could have important implications for how genetic information might be used by sporting organisations, which is a further reason for the need for sporting organisations to recognise the broader implications of gene doping policy. This argument is even more persuasive when one considers the state of sport ethics in relation to anti-doping policy. Sport ethics is already subservient to medical ethics to the extent that, what is ethically acceptable in sport relating to drug enhancement and doping is contingent upon what is ethically acceptable in medicine. Indeed, the policy statements concerning gene doping precisely reflect the ethical norm in medicine presently.

In response, sport ethicists might argue that this situation is inappropriate. Sport does not operate on the same kinds of norms and rules of broader society and, as such, it should not be held hostage to ethical guidelines in medical ethics. On this basis, the aim of sport ethicists would be to problematise sport as a moral practice, not medicine. Consequently, the application of medical ethical arguments in the case of genetic modification in sport is not as relevant as sports ethical arguments about what, for example, constitutes the 'good game'. Thus, even though sporting practices are constituted by what is medically acceptable, the critical question for sports ethicists would be whether or not they should be. If sport ought not be restricted by what is medically ethical, then conclusions about genetic modification in sport might be quite different.

VARIED INTERESTS, VARIED ARGUMENTS

To understand the context within which opinions about GM in sport are made by the IOC and WADA, it is necessary to recognise the historical legacy of anti-doping, drugs, and the evolution of policy in this area. The modern debate about doping emerged in the mid-1960s, as a result of some fatal incidents in competitive sport. Of particular importance was the death of English cyclist Tommy

Simpson, whose enduring image is in the Tour de France in 1967, during which he collapsed and later died. Since then, the IOC Medical Commission has worked to eradicate drugs from sport, though the consistency and logical basis of their policy have been questioned. For example, gender tests – widely recognised as lacking in scientific credibility and sexually prejudicial – have remained a part of Olympic doping tests until the Sydney 2000 Olympic Summer Games and even now have not been completely eliminated.

While the IOC Medical Commission has been able to maintain a relatively clean image throughout, the IOC was recently accused of corruption in its Olympic business dealings, where IOC members were alleged to have taken bribes to influence their voting decisions in regard to which cities were awarded the Olympic Games. The scandals of 1999, revealed in relation to the 2002 Salt Lake Olympic Winter Games bid process, were significant as they contrasted with the supposedly high morals of Olympism, the underlying philosophy of the Olympic Movement.[7] During the past five years, the IOC has been engaged in a process of reform, whereby it is endeavouring to distance itself from the morally corrupt past and appear socially responsible, financially transparent, and morally credible. It would be naïve to assume that such values and the desire for image-control do not encompass the IOC Medical Commission. Indeed, for many years there were some concerns about the IOC Medical Commission leading the anti-doping movement. Various critics have argued that the IOC has paid only lip service to the doping problem and has invested relatively few funds into combating the problem. Partly for this reason, in 1999, a new international doping body emerged, the World Anti-Doping Agency (WADA). This new organisation continues to retain close links with the IOC. Its Chairman, Richard Pound, was formerly on the Executive Board of the IOC and is credited with having saved the Olympic Movement from financial bankruptcy on more than one occasion. Also, the IOC has funded WADA in its entirety for the initial three years. Since 2002, the IOC has funded 50 per cent of WADA's operating budget, the remaining 50 per cent to be given by governments around the world. However, in 2001, circumstances emerged to suggest that not all governmental organisations had confidence in the new agency. For example, in Europe, the European Union was supposed to pay the share of all European Community countries. Yet, the Chair of the Cultural Commission (which includes sport), Vivian Reding, was unhappy with the transparency and hierarchy of WADA, concluding that the EU would be unable to make its financial commitment.

Presently, WADA seems on course to rectify these challenges, though it seems reasonable to say that they have hindered WADA's progress considerably in the past few years. Moreover, one might argue that there remains an important question to be asked about the infrastructure of anti-doping. I have attempted to suggest here that this infrastructure must now broaden itself beyond the traditional connections between sports and governments to encompass policy groups concerned with genetic technology more broadly. Without this additional layer of debate and without the broader contextualisation of sport policy about genetics, sports run the risk of marginalising themselves from changing social values about genetic technology. Moreover, they risk developing a policy that is inconsistent with the legal and moral concerns of the genetically modified athlete.

CONCLUSION: WHOEVER SAID IT SHOULD BE CALLED 'GENE DOPING'?

Presently, the emerging perspective in sport is to ensure gene doping does not become a method of performance enhancement for athletes This attempt to 'prevent' is certainly a departure from much of what has become the legacy of anti-doping policy, where policy has been largely 'reactive' rather than 'proactive' due largely to the difficulty of foreseeing what kinds of doping methods would emerge. However, it still remains unclear whether this approach will be informed by a critical reading of medical ethics.

While it would be an advance in anti-doping policy formation to re-visit core values of sport, this is not sufficient. This critique must also take place in the context of core medical values, which are problematised by the emergence of this new technology. Thus, it is not even clear that the old ethical principles of autonomy, justice, beneficence and non-maleficience are still effective in the context of the new genetics. I do not suggest that sport ethics should be subservient to medical ethics. Rather, it is to acknowledge that the process of argumentation within these distinct subjects borrows from similar methodologies and uses similar concepts. For example, the concepts of naturalness, personhood, humanness, normalcy, autonomy, and integrity are all discussed in great depth both in sport ethics and bioethics, though very rarely have the two disciplines sought to inform each other's respective analysis. Second, it is necessary to recognise that gene doping is not only a problem for sports authorities. It is not only the case that athletes might seek to use gene doping as a means of performance enhancement. Rather, it is also realistic to expect genetically modified humans to seek sport as a means by which they might prosper. Consequently, sporting authorities are not only dealing with athletes who are trying to cheat. They are also dealing with individuals who have been modified for non-sporting reasons, but who might be particularly gifted for sport for this reason. As well, decisions made about the use of gene doping in sport cannot be divorced from the social context within which they are situated. If specific forms of genetic modification are considered socially acceptable, then it might not be sufficient to maintain their prohibition from use in sport.

Finally, sporting authorities would do well to consider how best to describe the technology of gene doping. Indeed, the whole notion of gene doping seems un-satisfactory and unhelpful, as it creates a sense of how this technology must be evaluated, which limits the possibility of it being revised. Sporting authorities cannot approach the problem expecting only to deal with so-called 'cheats' who are deemed to be flouting sporting rules and values. This is not an argument for accepting gene transfer technology in sport at any cost. Rather, it recognises as of the utmost importance that the kind of discourse that this problem requires cannot be one that places neat and tidy policy-making ahead of the messy philosophising and ethical reasoning that must inform policy. Further work must seek to explain 'performance' in sport and reconcile this notion in the context of a range of performance modifiers, such as equipment, genetics, and doping methods (Miah and Eassom, 2002). Without this broader conceptualisation, sports risk limiting the ethics of sport to a political agenda that misrepresents how people value sport and biotechnology in the twenty-first century.

ACKNOWLEDGEMENTS

Sections of this chapter are reprinted from Miah (2003), © Council of Europe, and Miah (2004). Reprinted here with permission.

NOTES

1 Although, sport has always featured as a central example in a number of ethical papers on medical technology.
2 For an overview of this coverage, see the website 'Genetically Modified Athletes' at http://www.GMathletes.net
3 The distinction between 'safe' and 'possible' in science is an intriguing one. It would appear that genetic modification for sport is possible, though because it is not yet considered to be sufficiently safe, it is, therefore, considered to be impossible, though this is obviously not a coherent position. It appears that the intention of this perspective is to demonstrate that, even though there is a chance that genetic modification for athletes could result in some benefit to performance, it is highly unlikely and highly risky because there are no studies to validate the reliability of such experiments.
4 It will be of interest to note that the US President's Council on Bioethics has been criticised for spending too much time considering the ethical implications of technologies that are not yet real. For similar reasons, one might argue that the discussion about genetic enhancement in sport is reflective of an imagined ethical debate, which thus, lacks social value or importance. However, in this case, there is considerable disagreement as to how gene doping will emerge, which seems to justify debate.
5 This, of course, is a tricky position to sustain, since one can fully consent to knowing that the risks are uncertain and accept that level of risk.
6 While I suggest that this is a helpful and constructive way of approaching the matter, it might also be interpreted as a weakness, given the specificity of sports law.
7 Importantly, we must distinguish between the corruption of the Olympic committee and the corruption of the Olympic movement. The former was questioned in the 1999 scandals and it might be argued that the Olympic movement is particularly vulnerable to corruption because of its organisational structure and political value. However, this does not tell us anything about the state of Olympic values.

REFERENCES

Anderson, O. (2000) 'Now science is getting to the long and the short of how genes influence performance', *Peak Performance*, available at http://www.pponline.co.uk/encyc/0524.htm
Australia Law Reforms Commission (2003) ALRC 96: Essentially Yours.

Barton-Davis, E.R., Shoturma, D.I. *et al.* (1998) 'Viral Mediated Expression of Insulin-Like Growth Factor I Blocks the Aging-Related Loss of Skeletal Muscle Function', *Proceedings of the National Academy of Sciences, USA*, 95(December): 15603–7.

Brull, D., Dhamrait, S. *et al.* (2001) 'Bradykinin B2BKR Receptor Polymorphism and Left-Ventricular Growth Response', *The Lancet*, 358(October 6): 1155–6.

Clarey, C. (2001) 'Chilling New World: Sports and Genetics', *International Herald Tribune*, 26 Jan.

Gayagay, G., Yu, B. *et al.* (1998) 'Elite Endurance Athletes and the ACE I Allele – The Role of Genes in Athletic Performance', *Human Genetics*, 103(1): 48–50.

Goldspink, G. (2001) 'Gene Expression in Skeletal Muscle', *Biochemical Society Transactions*, 30: 285–90.

International Olympic Committee (2001) Press Release: IOC Gene Therapy Working Group – Conclusion. Lausanne, International Olympic Committee: available at http://www.olympic.org/uk/news/publications/press_uk.asp?release=179

Leiden, J.M. (2000) 'Human Gene Therapy: The Good, the Bad, and the Ugly', *Circulation Research* 86: 923.

Lin, J., Wu, H. *et al.* (2002) 'Transcriptional Co-activator PGC-1 Drives the Formation of Slow-Twitch Muscle Fibres', *Nature*, 418: 797–801.

Longman, J. (2001) 'Pushing the Limits: Getting the Athletic Edge May Mean Altering Genes', *The New York Times*, available at http://www.nytimes.com/2001/05/11/sports/11GENE.html

Miah, A. (2003) 'Gene-Doping: Sport, Values and Bioethics', in J. Glasa (ed.) *The Ethics of Human Genetics*, Strasburg, Council of Europe, pp. 171–80.

Miah, A. (2004) *Genetically Modified Athletes: Biomedical Ethics, Gene Doping and Sport*. London and New York: Routledge.

Miah, A. and Eassom, S.B. (eds) (2002) *Sport Technology: History, Philosophy & Policy*. Oxford: Elsevier Science.

Montgomery, H., Marshall, R. *et al.* (1998) 'Human Gene for Physical Performance', *Nature*, 393(21 May): 221–2.

Montgomery, H., Clarkson, P. *et al.* (1999) 'Angiotensin-converting-enzyme gene insertion/deletion polymorphism and response to physical training', *The Lancet*, 353 (February 13): 541–5.

Pérusse, L., Rankinen, T. *et al.* (2003) 'The Human Gene Map for Performance and Health-Related Fitness Phenotypes: The 2002 Update', *Medicine & Science in Sports & Exercise*, 35(8): 1248–64.

Plata, R., Cornejo, A. *et al.* (2002) 'Angiotensin-Converting-Enzyme Inhibition Therapy in Altitude Polycythaemia: A Prospective Randomised Trial', *The Lancet*, 359(9307): 663–6.

Powell, D. (2001) 'Spectre of Gene Doping Raises its Head as Athletes See Possibilities', *The Times*, 29 November.

Svensson, E.C., Black, H.B. *et al.* (1997) 'Long-term Erythropoietin Expression in Rodents and Non-Human Primates Following Intramuscular Injection of a Replication-Defective Adenoviral Vector', *Human Gene Therapy*, 8(15): 1797–806.

Taylor, R.R., Mamotte, C.D.S. *et al.* (1999) 'Elite Athletes and the Gene for Angiotensin Converting Enzyme', *Journal of Applied Physiology*, 87: 1035–7.

U.S. President's Council on Bioethics (2002) *Session 4: Enhancement 2: Potential for Genetic Enhancements in Sports*. Washington, DC, The President's Council on Bioethics: available at http://www.bioethics.gov/200207/session4.html

Williams, A.G., Rayson, M.P. *et al.* (2000) 'The ACE Gene and Muscle Performance', *Nature*, 403(10 February): 614.

World Anti-Doping Agency (2002) Press release: WADA Conference Sheds Light on the Potential of Gene Doping. New York, World Anti-Doping Agency: available at http://www.wada-ama.org.

World Anti-Doping Agency (2003) *Prohibited Classes of Substances and Prohibited Methods*. Lausanne: WADA.

Part II

The genetic enhancement of athletes

5   Genetic engineering and elitism in sport

Torbjörn Tännsjö

INTRODUCTION

The point of departure of this chapter is two observations, one rather common-place, and the other somewhat controversial. The first and commonplace observation is that many of us tend to admire the winners in elitist sport com-petitions. The second, and more controversial, is that there is something not quite right about this admiration. After having briefly indicated why I hold the latter opinion, I will discuss what kind of impact genetic engineering (enhance-ment) in sport would have on our admiration for the winners. I will argue that it would mean that what is problematic about our admiration would disappear. Hence, genetic engineering (enhancement) within sport is something we ought to welcome.

ELITISM

There is no denying that elitist sport, as the kind of cultural phenomenon we are now so familiar with, presupposes elitist values in society. It is because we admire the winners of the games that a great deal of money is allocated to the games. We watch them on television, we pay (indirectly) for the advertisements that are communicated through them, and so forth. This may seem pretty harmless, but my considered opinion is that it is not as harmless as it seems. What, then, is so bad about this kind of admiration? The problem, I conjecture, is that our enthusiasm for the winners has another side to it: contempt for those who lose, i.e., contempt for weakness. And contempt for weakness is at the heart of the Nazi ideology.

Nationalism, or chauvinism, or even racism, has sometimes been thought of as a defining trait of the Nazi ideology. However, in his seminal book, *Our Contempt for Weakness*, Harald Ofstad has argued – convincingly, it seems to me – that the nationalism and racism of the Nazis were only contingent facts.[1] Certainly, Hitler put the German nation before all other nations. And he put the so-called Aryan race before all other races. However, the hard core of Nazism was different; the hard core of Nazism was a contempt for weakness. This is shown by Hitler's reaction when the Third Reich was defeated. In Hitler's own opinion, the defeat showed, not that there was something basically wrong with the Nazi ideology, but that there was something basically wrong with the German nation, perhaps even with the Aryan race. The German nation had certainly proved to be weak rather than strong. So eventually Hitler came to feel contempt for it.[2]

How, then, does contempt for weakness enter our view of elitist sports competitions? Let me briefly recapitulate – and clarify – an argument I have put forward elsewhere. My argument depends on a crucial premise. It is certainly one thing to admire the person who wins the victory, who shows off as the strongest, but another thing to feel contempt for those who do not win (and turn out to be weak). The premise crucial to my argument is the conjecture that, by doing the one thing, we cannot help but do the other. This is how I think things actually are. When we celebrate and admire the winner, we cannot help but feel contempt for those who do not win. Admiration for the winner and contempt for the loser are only two sides of the same Olympic medal.

This is not to say that those who win the contest feel contempt for those who don't. It is one thing to compete and to want to win, and quite a different thing to admire, as a third party, the winner. My argument relates to those who view sports, not to those who perform. Those who perform may well consider other competitors as colleagues. They may feel that they are doing their job, and that is it. The winner may well feel respect for the loser. Or, the winner may entertain other feelings. It is not part of my project to speculate about this. My argument does not relate to the responses of the athletes; it relates to our responses as viewers to what they are doing. We, who comprise the public viewing the sports events, are the ones who admire the winner and feel contempt for the loser. If we are sincere in our admiration, and we often are, we cannot help but feel contempt for the losers. For simple phenomenological reasons we would be inconsistent if we did not feel any kind of contempt for the losers, once we sincerely admire the winner.

To see why this is so we ought to think critically about why we admire those who excel in the Olympics. Our feeling is based on a value judgement. Those who win the game, if the competition is fair, are excellent, and their excellence makes them valuable, which is why we admire them. Their excellence is, in an obvious manner, based on the strength or speed they exhibit in the competition. It is really that strength or speed they exhibit that we admire. And the strength they exhibit is 'strength' in a very literal sense of the word.

But our value terms are comparative. So, if we see a person as especially valuable, because of his or her excellence, and if that excellence is a manifestation of strength (in a very literal sense), then this must mean that other people, who do not win in a fair competition, those who are comparatively weak, are less valuable. The most natural feeling associated with this value judgement is – contempt. It is expressed in the popular saying: 'Being second is being the first among losers.'

These values, I submit, are false values. We make a moral mistake when we cheer for the winners. And the mistake we make has to do with the fact that the characteristic we admire in the winners, their strength, is a mere result of the genetic lottery. Those who win are not responsible for the strength they exhibit and that we admire.

It is certainly true that it takes not only a proper genetic constitution, but a lot of training as well, to become the winner in the 100 metres sprint final in the Olympics. However, many people are prepared to train enough to win, but only one person has the capacity to transform all the effort into a suitable physical constitution, which will provide complete success: the one with the best genotype will also produce the best phenotype. At least this must certainly be true in those sports where simple quality is enough to guarantee success.

Is it really a mistake to admire someone for something over which he or she could not exercise any choice? I think it is. From a utilitarian point of view, it is rather obvious that there is no point in praising someone for his or her natural endowments. Such praise makes no difference. And the corresponding blame expressed to the less talented will certainly do much harm.

Even a Kantian such as John Rawls would concur with this view. This is what Rawls has to say:

> Perhaps some will think that the person with greater natural endowments deserves those assets and the superior character that made their development possible. Because he is more worthy in this sense, he deserves the greater advantages that he could achieve with them. This view, however, is surely incorrect. It seems to be one of the fixed points of our considered judgments that no one deserves his place in the distribution of native endowments, any more than one deserves one's initial starting place in society.[2]

But even if our value judgement is mistaken, must we feel contempt for those who are less successful (valuable)? Can we not just admire them less?

I think not. For there are normative aspects of the notion as well. Those who are less valuable have to stand back when some good (and evils) are distributed. And when resources are scarce, treating one person well is tantamount to treating another person badly. In a sports situation, this is clearly so. The setting is competitive; the gold medals (and the money and reputation that go with them) are scarce resources.

This is not to say that, once we cheer for the winners, we must feel that those who are weak should be punished for their weakness, but the difference between punishment, and neglect, in a comparative setting, is, once again, merely verbal. If we were positively to condemn those who are weak, we would add insult to injustice; we need not do that when we cheer for the winners, but the injustice we do is bad enough as it is.

This is not to say that there are no virtues. Virtues are desirable character traits. We can distinguish between traits of personality, which are basically congenital and genetically determined, on the one hand, and, on the other, traits of character, which are of our own making. A virtuous person may very well be praised. There is a point in praising him or her, since this may encourage others to develop the same kind of character traits. And people who behave badly towards others may well be despised for this reason and this may teach them a lesson. There is a point in distributing praise and blame in this manner, since doing so may make a difference. It can make a difference since the target of this kind of praise and blame is a moral characteristic, a characteristic that we can adopt or develop if we decide to do so. Our moral character is open to change. However, there is no similar point in praising a person for the personality traits he or she exhibits, such as strength (or beauty), since strength (or beauty), in the relevant sense, is not a moral quality. Strength or the capacity for it, like physical beauty, is genetically determined, and hence it is not up to us to gain strength, if we do not possess the genes for it.

Obviously, there is no point in praising a person for his or her good genes. But, in effect, this is what we do when we cheer for the winner. We cheer for the strength he or she has exhibited, certainly, and not for his or her genes (we do not think about them). But when we cheer for his or her strength, we make a moral mistake. We treat the winner as if he or she were responsible for that strength, and we forget about its origin. If we were to contemplate its origin, we would have difficulties with our admiration. But we do not contemplate the origin of the strength exhibited, which is why we get carried away.

All this means that, when we cheer for the winner of the Olympic Games, we approach the core of the Nazi ideology. The idea that strength is a proper reason for admiration, the very idea that underlies our fascination for the winners of sports events, is one we cannot truthfully deny that we entertain, but it is an idea that we ought to resist.[3]

GENETIC ENGINEERING

Genetic engineering will soon be a possibility in sport. I will not go into specifics here, since this has been done in other contributions to this volume. I will assume that, eventually, very radical kinds of genetic enhancement of physical characteristics crucial to success in sport will be available, without going into detail. The reason for not going into detail is that, being a philosopher and not a scientist, I have no expertise in the field. Let me just assume that it will be possible genetically to design simple characteristics, such as the capacity for oxygen uptake, muscular volume, elasticity and strength, and so forth. Or, perhaps more plausibly, let us assume that methods will be available so that it will be possible to control crucial and strategic genes, allowing us to make people physically strong, irrespective, more or less, of their genetic constitution (provided it is not abnormal). I then want to investigate whether the putative fact that the winners will come to possess the (crucial) characteristics they do, not because they are winners in nature's genetic lottery, but because they have been genetically designed to this effect, means that we may view elitist sport in a more relaxed way. Does it mean that our admiration for the winners need no longer be of a fascistoid bent? It seems to me that this question must be answered in the affirmative.

Crucial to my argument to the effect that our contempt for weakness is fascistoid in nature is the assumption that those for whom we feel contempt, those who exhibit weakness, cannot do anything about this. By feeling contempt for their weakness, we feel contempt for them, and by expressing this contempt, even if indirectly, by cheering for those who are strong, we express contempt for those who are not strong. It is like celebrating the winners of a beauty contest while despising those who cannot, for natural reasons, compete.

However, if those who win the Olympic Games do so because of a clever choice of natural characteristics, or if those who win the beauty contest do so because of an artistically clever choice of physical characteristics, then we need not say that, by cheering for the winner and being less enthusiastic over those who lose, we express contempt for the losers. We now are celebrating a product, not a person. This is similar to great achievements in science and art. We may respect these achievements, without admiring those who have produced them. And we know that many of those who did not make great contributions to science and art may have been just as skilled as those who did but the latter were simply luckier.

It may certainly be objected that, even if the strength we admire in the winners of sports contests came to be found in those who had decided to develop a certain kind of physical strength, not those who were born with the right genes, there is still something strange about our fascination with strength.[4] The same can be said about beauty, of course. But it seems to me that, even if our fascination with strength and beauty is in some sense very superficial, the nasty implications of it tend to go away, once strength and beauty are something we can decide to adopt, or not to adopt, for ourselves. In particular, this would mean that the gender implications of the idea that a man should be strong and a woman beautiful would wither.

My comparison with what goes on in science and art may be questioned on the grounds that it is unfair. Is the situation in science and art the same as in sport? I think there is a crucial difference. There is no denying that, sometimes, there is something close to what happens within sport also found in science and art. Some people tend to admire the great scientist or the outstanding artist, not their accomplishments. And there may be prizes given for this reason as well. Scientists and artists may be treated as geniuses. To the extent that this is done, it is no better than what takes place in the sport context. However, when prizes are given in science and sport, what we express our fascination with may, and should, if we want to avoid the kind of criticism put forward here, be the fruitful scientific theories and the fantastic artistic products, to which we wish to draw attention. We value fruitful theories and great art, of course, but this valuation is not a moral one. We take pleasure in these theories and these pieces of art, that is all there is to it. And this kind of emotion is quite innocuous.

Now, if genetic enhancement became a standard part of sport, the difference between science and art would wither. We would still admire the strength exhibited by the winning athlete. But his or her physical constitution would now be something he or she had decided to adopt. By the prize given to the winner, we would express our fascination with this natural product – which would be a joint product of the athlete him or herself and the pharmaceutical company that had developed the method the athlete (or his or her parents) chose to use. So there seems to be a very good reason to welcome genetic engineering within sport – just like ordinary doping, at least to the extent that it means a levelling out of congenital differences between competitors.

BUT IS IT FAIR?

Both ordinary doping and genetic enhancement have been objected to on the grounds that they give unfair advantages to those who resort to them. To the extent that they are prohibited, this is true in a very literal sense. To resort to them, when they are prohibited, means cheating. However, why prohibit them in the first place?

Behind the idea that they should be prohibited lies an interest in having genetically determined factors settling the outcome of the competitions, it seems to me. And to the extent that this interest forms part of the ethos of elitist sport, both doping and genetic enhancement are at variance with this ethos; they provide an unfair advantage. There is a long history in sports testifying to this fact. There was a time when training was looked upon with suspicion. This would give an unfair advantage to those who trained. No one questions training today, and all athletes engage in it. Why? Because it was impossible to check whether people had trained or not. So the idea was then that, if everyone trained, then everyone had an equal chance of winning, and the genetic constitution would be decisive, not the amount of training. Then came a time when massive training, on a professional basis, was condemned; I can vividly recollect the disdain with which swimmers from Eastern Germany were regarded by the Western media in the 1960s. These days are also gone. Today all successful athletes train on a professional and scientific basis. Why? Once again because there was no way of telling who had trained on a regular and normal basis and who had trained excessively. To the extent that all have the same resources at their disposal (an ideal we are far from realising, of course, because of social differences and differences between nations), the competitions remain fair. And, once again, if all the athletes train excessively, then the genetic disposition becomes decisive for who will win and who will lose.

But if training, even on a professional and scientific basis is all right, then why not accept doping as well, at least so long as the drugs used are not especially dangerous to the user? This would certainly mean a change of the ethos of elitist sport. But why not change the ethos? As a matter of fact, I think sport is on the verge of giving in to doping. The reason for doing so is, once again, that there is no way of ascertaining who has used prohibited drugs and who hasn't. If we were to permit all kinds of performance-enhancing drugs, we would no longer need to entertain the uneasy suspicion that the winner had used prohibited drugs and managed to get away with it. We could then watch the games in a more relaxed manner.

If we were to accept doping within sport, would this mean that, once again, fair conditions for the competition had been restored? Would it mean that those who have the best genetic set-up would win? This is far from certain and this is probably why both doping and genetic enhancement are so controversial. To some extent the use of performance-enhancing drugs may mean that those who are less well equipped genetically will catch up on those who are better equipped. And according to the existing ethos of sport, this is not fair. There is a much-publicised example of this. Throughout his career in the 1960s, the Finnish cross-country skier Eero Mäntyranta was suspected of blood doping because his red blood count was 20 per cent higher than that of other athletes. Thirty years later, scientists tested 200 members of his family and discovered that fifty of them, including Mäntyranta himself, were born with a rare genetic mutation that causes an increase in oxygen-rich red blood cells. This mutation, in the heyday of his career, made Mäntyranta almost invincible. Today his less genetically endowed competitors could, in order to catch up with him, have resorted to EPO-doping. Or, when he was active, his competitors could have resorted to old-fashioned blood doping. Many people would think that this was unfair. My strong feeling is that this kind of sentiment may explain why the resistance to doping is more stubborn than the opposition ever was to training, or even to systematic training.

But does this opposition to doping rest on a sound moral foundation? Would it have been unfair if Mäntyranta's main competitors had had the same red blood count as he had? I think not. The very notion of justice entertained within sport must be flawed, then. So there are very good reasons indeed to change the ethos of elitist sport in precisely this respect. The very idea that natural talent, that congenital strength, that genetically determined personality traits, should lead to victory and praise, is deeply unsound.

It is difficult to avoid this notion of justice within sport. We all tend to cling to it, it seems, but eventually, due to the rapid medical development it is now becoming obsolete. Here science seems to conspire with morality in a fruitful manner that promises moral progress within future sport.

DOES GENETIC ENGINEERING THREATEN THE DIGNITY OR AUTONOMY OF ATHLETES?

Elitist sport has in many ways become an important cultural phenomenon, and the role of large corporations in sport events is of crucial importance to the very existence of this phenomenon, as we know it today. This has brought with it all sorts of tensions within the sports movement. Commercial interests are in conflict with nationalistic ones, professionalism is in conflict with old and deeply entrenched ideals of sportsmanship, and so on. And yet, much of the original ethos of the sports movement remains, in a more modern and up-to-date form, even when it comes to events such as the Olympic Games. However, the impact of pharmaceutical companies, designing all sorts of characteristics crucial to excellence in sport, would mean something qualitatively new, a step towards a radically new ethos. There is no comparison, in this respect, with the impact of big business in sports. The introduction of genetic engineering in sport would mean that sports competitions would become similar to competitions in Formula 1. There are certainly people driving the cars, but more important than their skill is the design of the car. The same would be true of sports events in general. The athletes would be conducting their bodies in the arena, but their bodies would be designed by the pharmaceutical companies. And our cheers for the winners would, to a large extent, concern the products created by these companies (in cooperation with the athletes, of course, who are supposed to be taking care of their bodies, tending them, keeping them in good shape, and so on, just the way that a good Formula 1 driver takes care of his car). Not even hard training need be necessary in the future, if some of the most utopian prophecies are borne out by realities. This is how one of the leading experts in the field described the future: 'With the basic knowledge in hand, it now may be possible to develop a pill that pumps up muscle cells without all that exercise', said Dr R. Saunders Williams, Dean of the Duke University School of Medicine, North Carolina, and senior author of a study appearing in the journal *Science*, on the role of PGC-1 for health-related muscle adaptations.[5] Some may feel that this is in some way objectionable. Some may feel that, by allowing pharmaceutical companies to design winners of sports events, and even to liberate the athletes from the need to resort to hard training, we are allowing pharmaceutical companies to use human beings as mere guinea pigs. Is there something in this kind of accusation? I think not.

First of all, it is far from obvious that it is wrong to use another human being as a mere means. The assertion that this is wrong is certainly crucial in one kind of ethical theory, advocated most famously by Immanuel Kant, but this ethical theory is controversial. Be that as it may, however, let us just for the sake of the argument assume that it is wrong to use a human being as a mere means. We then have to query whether genetic engineering would have this effect. Is it true that pharmaceutical companies, who design winning characteristics for athletes, would use the athletes as mere means? This does not strike me as true.

First of all, even if a certain pharmaceutical company enrols only some athletes in its 'stable', providing them with the desired characteristics only on the assumption that the genetically modified athletes would in so many ways do their best to promote the reputation of the company, entering into this kind of contract would have to be a voluntary move, at least if it takes place in a reasonably liberal society. So, while it is true that the company does use the athlete as a means, it is hardly true to say that it would use the athlete as a mere means. There must be something in the deal for the athlete as well; otherwise he or she would not have entered into the bargain. And it is obvious that there would be something for the athlete as well, in terms both of money and fame – provided the company is successful.

Second, the fact that a person has him or herself chosen all sorts of physical characteristics (traits of personality), seems to render true a crucial tenet of existentialist philosophy, to wit, that our physical existence precedes our personal one (our 'essence'). If this affects our degree of dignity or autonomy, it should mean that it will be increased, not that it is in any way threatened.

I have now taken for granted that the genetic therapy in question is somatic. What if it takes the form of germ-line intervention? What if the parents contract with pharmaceutical companies and choose physical characteristics for their children? Would this mean a threat to the dignity or autonomy of the children?

Once again, I think we have to answer the question in the negative. These children would simply find that they were born with certain characteristics that are there through no choice of theirs. But this has up to now been the normal human condition. No one has complained that this means a threat to our dignity or autonomy. I see no difference in a case where the parents choose and a case where the natural genetic lottery is free to operate unperturbed by human intervention. However, once it becomes possible to design the characteristics of your children, parents become responsible for their children in a new manner. This is a responsibility they cannot avoid. Also the decision not to use genetic engineering, once it is possible, is also a decision the parents must take responsibility for.

Interestingly enough, a Kantian such as John Rawls finds nothing to object to in principle against genetic engineering (enhancement). This is how he speculates about the future with respect to genetic engineering in general (but with no reference to sport in particular): 'We might conjecture that in the long run, if there is an upper bound on ability, we would eventually reach a society with the greatest equal liberty, the members of which enjoy the greatest equal talents.'[6]

If he is correct in assuming that there is an upper bound on (physical) ability, then genetic engineering promises to provide a kind of natural justice (equality). However, more plausibly, there is no obvious upper bound when it comes to physical strength, and the results of genetic enhancement, together with the use of new and safe forms of doping, will provide us with a series of astonishing accomplishments. There will be so many ways of rendering true the Olympic motto 'Citius, altius, fortius' (faster, higher, stronger).

Genetic engineering would also mean better chances of sexual equality within sport. If women, for example, on average, have less muscular volume than men, this can be corrected through genetic engineering, and equal opportunities can be provided to both sexes. One time a women happens to win, the next time a man, this all depends on how inventive the scientists are who are hired by the pharmaceuticals taking care of respective athlete.

Note also that, if a child is not satisfied with the characteristic in question, there may be a way to correct nature, when somatic genetic intervention becomes common. And certainly, in a liberal society, the parents should not be free to bind their children before their birth into any contracts with pharmaceutical companies. Such a contract, struck by the parents on behalf of their (future) children, should be considered void in a liberal society.

WOULD GERM-LINE GENETIC ENGINEERING VIOLATE THE RIGHT TO BE BORN WITH A GENOME WHICH NO ONE HAS MANIPULATED?

It has sometimes been held that germ-line genetic enhancement means that the right to a genome that no one has tampered with is thwarted. The parliamentary session of the Council of Europe suggested on 26 January 1982, in its Recommendation No. 934, that the right to life article in the Convention for the Protection of Human Rights and Fundamental Freedoms should be understood to imply that a right exists to a genome with which no one has tampered. Such interventions have indeed later been prohibited, in the recent Convention on Human Rights and Biomedicine (ETS No. 164) adopted by the Council of Europe. Article 13 it stipulates: 'An intervention seeking to modify the human genome may only be undertaken for preventive, diagnostic or therapeutic purposes and only if its aim is not to introduce any modification in the genome of any descendants.' However, I don't think this argument from a rights-based philosophy fares any better than the denontological one just discussed. Even if there are basic moral rights that moral agents hold in virtue of being moral agents (and this too is controversial, of course), the right to a genome with which no one has manipulated is not among them. To see this we need only distinguish between the following two cases.

First of all, if the intervention is small, and to the satisfaction of the person having been manipulated, there doesn't seem to be room for any complaint. A child has obtained a gene for a certain physical skill, say, with which the individual is satisfied – or at least indifferent. Then, nothing in principle seems to have gone wrong. Of course, if the manipulation is not to the satisfaction of the individual who has been manipulated, then there is room for complaint. But then the complaint is not a principled one, it is not directed against manipulation as such, but it should rather be directed against the nature and extent of the particular genetic intervention that has taken place. If the person is happy to use the acquired characteristic, or happy not to use it, then it seems to me obvious that no right of the child has been affected.

On the other hand, if the intervention is radical, so radical that, as a matter of fact, had it not taken place, the individual who exists as a result of it, would not have existed, and if the individual in question leads a good life, then, once again, there is no room for any complaint. After all, a complaint that the manipulation took place must mean, under the circumstances, that the person making the complaint would have preferred a situation where he or she did not exist at all.

There seem to be no principled arguments against allowing genetic intervention, either in society in general or in sport, then.[7] It also seems clear that, once radical medical advances become possible through, and only through, germ-line genetic therapy (such as genetic 'vaccinations' against diseases such as cancer, Alzheimer's, Parkinson, diabetes, and so on), there will be no way of stopping such a development, all the ethical conventions to the contrary notwithstanding. And once such a development has started, for strictly medical reasons, it will be difficult to see why one should not put it also to other kinds of use, such as in sport. I think we ought to welcome such a development. This is not to say that genetic engineering in general may not come to pose problems to society and the individual, but I will not go into this general discussion here. Let it suffice to say that I believe there are responsible ways for society to respond to these challenges, reaping the fruits of these new medical technologies, while steering clear of the major dangers posed by them.[8]

THE FUTURE OF ELITIST SPORT

However, even if the effects of genetic engineering, both somatic and germ-line, may prove in the final analysis to be positive on a broad societal level, special problems may come to surface in sport. What if those who win the Olympic Games in some not too distant future are not winners in a natural genetic lottery, but genetically designed to do what they do? Would we still be prepared to stay up all night to watch them perform? Would we still be prepared to admire those who make the best achievements? Would we still be prepared to cheer for the winners?

I have earlier conjectured that we would not.[9] If this conjecture is correct, it means that genetic engineering threatens elitist sport as the kind of cultural phenomenon with which we are only too familiar. Some may find this sad. I am not among them. Since our admiration for the winners, and our fascination with elitist sport rest, if my argument is correct, on fascistoid evaluations, there is no reason to complain, if our interest withers. There are still so many ways of both taking part in, and viewing sport, in the form of sportsmanship, that we can very well do without elitist sport of the kind we now know.

However, I have become more suspicious about my earlier conjecture. It now seems to me that our interest in elitist sport may well come to survive the introduction of genetic enhancement of the athletes. After all, many people do take much interest in Formula 1 competitions. Future elitist sport would not be much different from that. As a matter of fact, it may be even more fascinating to watch athletes conducting their bodies than drivers driving their cars. The future achievements in sport may turn out to be extraordinary. And we do constantly demand more remarkable results in sport. Genetic engineering may be the means of providing what we want. So why not keep watching the show, why not stay up the night to find out which firm has produced the most talented athlete? Why not stay up and cheer for, not the winning person as such, but for the scientific achievement – the product – made by the pharmaceutical company in question?

It might be thought that if those who compete now are too different from us, we would no longer be able to identify with them. But this is not true. Today I realise that, no matter how hard I train, I will never be able to run a 100-metre sprint final anywhere near as fast as Ben Johnson or Carl Lewis did. However, when, in the future, I watch a final where the winner runs faster than 5 seconds,

I know that, had I decided to adopt the very same characteristics, I could have done so as well. The winner doesn't look like me, but looks can be changed!

I think, upon reflection, that a continued and even increased interest in elitist sport is what will be forthcoming if doping and genetic enhancements become standard parts of the business. But then, this is good news. For now our admiration has eventually taken a form that could stand up to critical moral scrutiny! We admire and respect not the athletes as such, but we feel a non-moral, purely aesthetic fascination, with the results of theirs and the drug companies' joint efforts.

This means that very distinction made above between traits of character, on the one hand, and traits of personality, on the other, tends to become a distinction without any difference. What has been taken to be congenital traits of personality, such as a capacity for physical strength (or intelligence) become more like traits of character, i.e., something we choose for ourselves (and for our children) through genetic modification. While an elitist sport contest today bears a great deal of similarity to a Miss World contest, where congenital talent is praised, it will in the future be more like a contest as to who-is-best-dressed-in the world. Even if I find values such as strength and beauty somewhat superficial, I have no moral objection to such contests.

CONCLUSION

The point of departure of my discussion was the observation that our admiration for those who win elitist sport contests is based on perverted moral values. We treat the winner as if he or she were responsible for the strength exhibited. We treat the winner as if he or she deserved our praise, but really he or she is a winner of the natural genetic lottery and doesn't deserve these natural endowments. Moreover, when we cheer for the winner, when we express our fascination with his or her strength or speed, we are trapped in a thinking that constitutes the core of the Nazi ideology: fascination for strength and contempt for weakness. However, if we know that those who win the gold medals have been genetically designed to do so, and if we know that they possess the physical characteristics they do through a free choice of their own, then this means that we can take a more relaxed view of elitist sport. Now there is no harm in cheering for the winner. By cheering for him or her, we congratulate the winner on his or her wise choice of characteristics, and we take pleasure in and are fascinated with these characteristics as such. Even if such fascination may be considered superficial, it is by no means evil.

NOTES

1   Harald Ofstad, *Our Contempt for Weakness* (Stockholm: Almqvist & Wiksell, 1989).
2   Ibid., p. 24.

3 I develop this argument more fully in 'Is Our Admiration for Sports Heroes Fascistoid?' in Torbjörn Tännsjö and Claudio Tamburrini (eds), *Values in Sports: Elitism, Nationalism, Gender Equality, and the Scientific Manufacture of Winners* (London and New York: E&FN Spon/Routledge, 2000), reprinted in William J. Morgan, Klaus V. Meier, and Angela Schneider (eds), *Ethics in Sport* (Champaign, IL: Kinetics, 2001).

4 I owe this observation to Anna-Karin Andersson, a research student in Stockholm.

5 Quoted in *Associated Press*, April 2002. I thank Professor Bengt Saltin for drawing my attention to this quoted passage.

6 *A Thory of Justice*, p. 108.

7 I defend this claim more fully in 'Should We Change the Human Genome?', *Theoretical Medicine*, 14, 1993: 231–47.

8 I discuss this general theme in my book *Coercive Care: The Ethics of Choice in Health and Medicine* (London and New York: Routledge, 1999). Cf. also my 'Human Genetics and the Nazi Spectre', *Monash Bioethics Review*, 18, 1999: 13–21.

9 'Is Our Admiration for Sports Heroes Fascistoid?', op. cit.

6 What's wrong with admiring athletes and other people?

Ingmar Persson

INTRODUCTION

The aim of this chapter is to examine Torbjörn Tännsjö's claim that we ought to welcome genetic engineering in sports because it will undercut our 'fascistoid' admiration of sport stars.[1] Tännsjö seems to think that this admiration is fascistoid because it is based on something – 'strength' – which is genetically determined and therefore outwith our responsibility. It is here argued that, though the fact that admiration for somebody is based on some property beyond responsibility makes admiration improper, it does not make it fascistoid. Even though they need involve no assumptions about responsibility, the emotions of attraction and repulsion can be fascistoid, if they block out concern for the well-being of people. Further, if genetic engineering were to put strength within the reach of responsibility, it would allow fascistoid tendencies to express themselves in the emotion of admiration, albeit if this engineering is used to level out human differences, there will be less scope for this emotion. It is also argued that the admiration of sport stars is only to a very limited extent admiration of them because of their strength. Finally, an argument is sketched that locates the immorality of fascistoid attitudes in their being fundamentally unjust.

In his provocative chapter in this volume, 'Genetic Engineering and Elitism in Sport'. Torbjörn Tännsjö argues that 'genetic engineering (enhancement) within sport is something we ought to welcome' because it will make 'what is problematic about our admiration' of winners in sports events 'disappear' (p. 57). This admiration is (morally) problematic, he claims, because it is 'of a fascistoid bent' (p. 60). It is of this bent for the reason that the idea that underlies it is that 'strength is a proper reason for admiration' (p. 60). 'Strength, or the capacity for it,' as he conceives it, 'is genetically determined, and hence it is not up to us to gain strength, if we do not possess the genes for it' (p. 60). But when we admire the winner, we treat him 'as if he was responsible for his strength' (p. 60) and forget about its genetic origin. Were we to contemplate this origin, 'we would have difficulties maintaining with our admiration' (p. 60).

If, however, it became possible to genetically design strength, our admiration would take 'a form that could stand up to critical moral scrutiny' (p. 68). We would no longer admire 'the athletes as such', but would 'feel a non-moral, purely aesthetic fascination' (p. 68) with a certain product . This product is the result of the choice of athletes among the ways of improving their physique offered by genetic technology.

In opposition to this, I shall contend that if our admiration of sports stars is fascistoid, it is not because it is based on a feature for which people are erroneously taken to be responsible. I will give examples of emotions that can be fascistoid, though they involve no such mistake. Since admiration is proper only if it is based on features for which the subjects are responsible, the development of genetic engineering would rather have the effect of making admiration of strength proper. It is another matter if genetic engineering could restrict the scope for such an emotion by affecting a levelling out of congenital differences between human beings (p. 62). This does not show that there is anything wrong with this emotion. I will end by giving an argument which reveals what is wrong with it. We will also see that the admiration of sport stars is only to a very limited extent an admiration of them because of their physical strength.

THE RELATION BETWEEN ADMIRATION AND CONTEMPT

Tännsjö apparently believes that in order to show that our admiration for the winners of sports events is of a fascist kind, he has to bring it home that there is 'another side to it: contempt for those who lose, i.e., contempt for weakness. And contempt for weakness is at the heart of the Nazi ideology' (p. 57). It is true that contempt is the other 'side' of admiration in the sense that it is the opposite of it. Logically to be a proper object of admiration, I think, someone must be worthy or deserving of praise, reward or some form of treatment that is good for this individual. Therefore, this individual must be superior in some valuable respect.[2] In contrast, those who are contemptible, i.e., worthy or deserving of blame and punishment, must be inferior in some respect of value or importance.

The pair admiration–contempt is the 'other-person' counterpart of pride and shame. What one is proud of is oneself, or somebody with whom one 'identifies' (such as a member of one's family or nation), whom one regards as worthy or deserving of praise or reward and, therefore, as superior in some valuable respect, and what one is ashamed of is oneself, or someone with whom 'identifies', whom one regards as worthy or deserving of blame and punishment and, so, as inferior in some valuable respect.

Now, in-between the superior and inferior, obviously there is to be found a group, members of which are neither superior or inferior, but only average. In order to feel admiration and contempt, we need a reference class whom those admired rise above and those despised fall below. Those in the reference class are neither admirable nor contemptible, but just average. This is, however, not Tännsjö's view. He seems to think that all but the most superior, the very best, are contemptible, for he writes that those 'who do not win in a fair competition, those who are comparatively weak, are less valuable. The most natural feeling associated with this value judgement is – contempt' (p. 58). Even those who end up second are construed as the objects of contempt.

This is implausible. The second-placed in, say, a sprint final may be almost as good as winner (in fact, he may in general be better, but end up second only because of a stroke of bad luck). In any event, he is normally superior to most of us in running capacity. Therefore, he is almost as admirable as the winner, rather than contemptible. In comparison to us, we couch potatoes, sitting watching the contest, he is quite superior. So, if we are going to despise anyone, we should despise ourselves rather than him or any other contestant. Moreover, according to this logic, we should despise more those who are handicapped or ill and for that reason even worse runners. They are the ones who are most inferior when it comes to running.

One reason why Tännsjö ends up in this extreme position is that he apparently equates feeling contempt for somebody with the negative state of merely withholding admiration of this person. He writes, for instance, that 'by expressing this contempt, even if indirectly, by cheering for those who are strong, we express contempt for those who are not strong' (p. 61), i.e., for those for whom we do not cheer. But this is no more plausible than saying that by expressing our love for the beloved, we 'indirectly' express our hatred of all those not embraced by our love! This is obviously false, however, since hatred is not to be identified with the mere absence of love.[3] I conclude, then, that Tännsjö builds his case for the admiration of strength being an fascistoid emotion on a very peculiar link to contempt for weakness.

WHAT IS THE FASCISTOID EMOTION OR EVALUATION?

I do not think, however, that it would damage Tännsjö's case were he to concede the possibility of having admiration of the strong without being contemptuous of the weak. For it is still true that admiration of the strong is the opposite of contempt for the weak, and it seems to me no less (and no more) plausible to claim that admiration of what is strong, healthy and fit for survival is distinctive or definitive of Fascism and Nazism than that contempt for the weak, sick and unfit is distinctive or definitive of it.

So, let us look at Tännsjö's reason for viewing contempt for weakness as fascistoid, taking it for granted that it holds, *mutatis mutandi*, for admiration of the strong: 'Crucial to my argument to the effect that our contempt for weakness is fascistoid in nature is the assumption that those whom we feel contempt for, those who exhibit weakness, cannot do anything about this' (p. 61). I agree that it is unjustifiable to be contemptuous of people because of some feature of theirs that they cannot do anything about (and have never been able to do anything about). This is connected with the point made earlier that to be a logically proper object of this emotion one must be worthy or deserving of blame or punishment, because one is inferior in some valuable respect. For one cannot be worthy or deserving of blame or punishment for being inferior, if one is not responsible for this inferiority. This is because if one is worthy or deserving of blame or punishment, it is just that one is blamed or punished. For instance, we do not feel contempt for people because they are dwarfs or crippled, as we realize that this is due to some congenital disease and not at all to any fault of theirs. It is unjust to blame and punish people for shortcomings they cannot help. Such shortcomings are rather something that makes compassion called for – or, if we are deficient in humanity – disgust and repulsion. Similarly, we do not admire people simply because they are tall, though we might find their height attractive and impressive, for we know they are not responsible for their height.

It may be objected that we say that we admire natural phenomena such as beautiful landscapes or sunsets. Yes, but here 'admire' cannot mean anything other than 'enjoy', 'take pleasure in' or 'be impressed by'. According to my analysis, there are two reasons why we cannot admire in the genuine sense for natural phenomena. (Note that we hardly say that we feel contempt for ugly natural phenomena, such as a forest ravaged by a fire.) First, for X to be a proper object of admiration, it must make sense to praise or reward X, or to treat X in a way that is good for it; otherwise, it makes no sense to say that X is deserving or worthy of such treatment. This implies, I think, that a proper object of admiration must be a sentient being. Second, since this object must be deserving or worthy of this treatment, it must be a responsible being, who is responsible for its superiority or inferiority.

Tännsjö apparently shares my view that if you are to be rightly admired because of some feature of yours, you must be responsible for having it, since otherwise you cannot deserve anything in virtue of it. For he argues:

> our admiration for those who win elitist sport contests is based on perverted moral values. We treat the winner as if he or she were responsible for the strength exhibited. We treat the winner as if he or she deserved our praise, but really he or she is a winner of the natural genetic lottery and doesn't deserve these natural endowments.
>
> (p. 68)

But it cannot be the fact, that admiration of some people because of their strength and contempt of others because of their weakness is admiration and contempt based on some characteristic for which they are not responsible, that makes these emotions fascistoid. Suppose you admire some people because of their kind-heartedness and this turns out to be a congenital trait. This would make your admiration mistaken (though you could still like or approve of these people because of their kind-heartedness), but it obviously does not make it fascistoid. So, the fact that this admiration is based upon properties for which people are mistakenly thought to be responsible cannot be enough to make it fascistoid.

Now consider some elitists who do not despise people whom they recognize to be weak, disabled and disfigured through bad luck, genetical or environmental, because they realize that this background makes contempt inappropriate. Instead they are repelled or disgusted by these invalids. Suppose further that this repulsion or disgust is so strong that these elitists think these invalids should be forgotten, perhaps even exterminated, not, however, because they think these invalids deserve it, but simply because their presence is a stain on society or the human species. That is, their 'aesthetic' disgust at these unfortunates is so strong that it overpowers or silences any concern that any humane person would feel for their suffering. This attitude to the invalids seems to me a no less suitable candidate for the epithet 'fascistoid' than does contempt for them. But it is not based on any mistaken belief to the effect that these invalids are responsible for their short-comings. Hence, this mistaken belief is not necessary for an attitude to be fascistoid.

What all this leads up to is the following conclusion. When people are despised because of some feature of theirs, such as their weakness, two evaluations are made of them. First, they are judged inferior or less valuable because of their weakness. Second, they are judged to be worth something negative, punishment, etc., in virtue of possessing this valueless feature of weakness, for which they are seen as responsible. Tännsjö suggests that a mistaken evaluation of the second sort is essential for a fascistoid attitude. My reasoning suggests that the first evaluation suffices if it is strong enough to silence concern for the well-being of the weak. The same holds, *mutatis mutandi*, for admiration. In other words, one's liking for strength is fascistoid if it is so strong that one excessively favours the interests of the strong.

This has severe consequences for Tännsjö's view that the introduction of genetic engineering of strength would allow our admiration of it to take 'a form that could stand up to critical moral scrutiny' (p. 68), that is, a form that is not fascistoid. For the introduction of this technique does not show that there is anything wrong with an excessive positive evaluation or liking of strength, which we have found to be fascistoid. Furthermore, by giving us the means to manipulate strength, genetic engineering would eliminate the objection to admiring strength to the effect that strength is nothing for which we are responsible. For it may now well be. Thus, our fascistoid inclinations may now express themselves in the attitude of admiration. The upshot is therefore exactly the opposite of what Tännsjö claims: genetic engineering of strength would underpin rather than undercut the foothold of admiration of strength which he takes to be fascistoid.

I conjecture that one reason why he fails to see this is that he believes – wrongly, as we have seen – that admiration of strength is fascistoid because it is admiration of something for which people are not responsible. So, if strength becomes something for which people are responsible, it would seem that admiration of it will no longer be fascistoid. But the objection to admiration of strength so long as it is of something for which we are not responsible is not that it is fascistoid, but that the logical conditions for admiration being proper are not fulfilled. If strength becomes something for which we are responsible, these conditions are fulfilled.

Tännsjö is also misled, I hypothesize, by a false dichotomy between admiration of 'athletes as such' and 'the non-moral, purely aesthetic fascination' with what they produce (p. 68). There is no 'either–or' but a 'both' here. As was remarked above, there are two evaluations involved when people are admired for some property of theirs, such as their strength: this property of theirs is valued and they are thought to be worth something in virtue of being responsible for having this valuable property. Contrary to what Tännsjö seems to believe, the introduction of large-scale genetic manipulation would not force a retreat from admiring people or thinking them worthy of something to a 'fascination' or evaluation of properties of theirs that underlie the admiration. Why should it when this manipulation rather increases that for which we are responsible? Moreover, this fascination could assume fascistoid proportions, as we have seen.

There is, however, a way in which large-scale genetic engineering could diasarm or render harmless fascistoid attitudes. As Tännsjö notes, it could bring about a levelling out of congenital differences between human beings (p. 62). There is in nature a terrible inequality and injustice as some are born with genes that predispose them to develop much stronger and healthier bodies than others. As a consequence, they will have longer and better lives. Genetic engineering in a future advanced state could be employed to decrease this inequality, not only by eliminating congenital diseases, but also by enhancing desirable traits. I agree with Tännsjö that this would be a salutary effect, making the world less genetically unjust. But one such salutary effect would not be to make our emotions of admiration and contempt less 'fascistoid'. Extensive genetic engineering could, however, decrease the scope for feeling these emotions, decrease the scope for fascistoid differentiation. For in a world in which people were more equal in assets, there would be less occasion to value some higher than others, that is, there would be less differentiation in respect of the first evaluation above.

While genetic engineering would give less opportunity for the exercise of fascistoid differentiation, it would not show what is wrong or immoral about it. Below I shall, however, sketch a metaphysical argument which does precisely that, by showing that this differentiation leads to distributions that are unjust or unfair. This argument is to the effect that, ultimately, people are not responsible for any of their more or less valuable features. If this is so, it follows that nobody deserves or is worthy of leading better lives than any other and, thus, that it would be unjust if some lead better lives than others. But this is precisely what fascistoid differentiation would lead to.

THE GROUNDS FOR ADMIRATION OF SPORT STARS AND THE POSSIBILITY OF IMPROVING THEM

I have so far gone along with Tännsjö's claim that we admire athletes because of their strength 'or the capacity for it'. But surely we do not admire people merely because they have a genetically determined capacity to develop a physique that would make them excellent at some sport. Suppose that they have this capacity but do nothing to exercise it. This may make us criticize them for wasting their gifts. Instead, we admire sport stars because they have brought off certain achievements, such as winning a contest or breaking a record.

This is similar to the situation in art and science. Here too we admire people, artists and scientists, because of their achievements. A difference is that in the latter case the achievement may be a long-lasting product – a painting, novel or scientific treatise – that outlives the producing of it. Admiration of sport stars is more akin to the admiration of artists in the performing arts, such as actors playing certain parts or musicians playing certain pieces of music. In both cases, people are admired because of certain performances they undertake.

In all probability, a certain genetic endowment is necessary to pull off an outstanding athletic performance. But clearly it is not sufficient: to win a major competition you obviously also have to invest in massive training and a healthy life-style. Therefore, there is a point in praising athletes for victories just as Tännsjö notes that there is a point in praising people for their 'traits of character', such as their moral virtues (p. 59). He remarks that the latter sort of admiration can be justified because it 'may make a difference' to future behaviour; it may encourage people to persevere with their standards of conduct. Similarly, praising winners may also make a difference to their future behaviour: it may motivate them to persevere with their hard, time-consuming training.

Nonetheless, no amount of training is enough on its own to make a successful athlete. You also need a certain genetic endowment, e.g., a supernormal capacity for oxygen uptake or certain skeletal or muscular features. But the same is true of success in the arts and science, for instance, no amount of diligent practice will make you a good pianist or ballet dancer, unless you have the right gift. Hence, if we conclude with Tännsjö, that admiration of successful athletes is for this reason improper – as long as 'strength' cannot be genetically designed – we should draw the same conclusion as regards artists and scientists.

Tännsjö may well accept this corollary for he writes that when artists and scientists are treated as geniuses, this 'is no better than what takes place in the sport context' (p. 61). His contention seems to be that we should only 'take pleasure in' what they produce, artworks, scientific theories, and so on. I shall come back to this claim, but there is no denying that the majority of us in fact admire great artists and scientists (and despise bad ones),[4] just as we admire great athletes.

Thus, strength – by which Tännsjö means physical strength – is not enough to make anyone qualify as an object of athletic admiration. But in the case of many sports, physical strength to any higher degree than normal is not even a necessary condition for success. Table tennis, archery, fencing and billiards are cases in point. Thus, even if admiration because of some performance for which physical strength is a necessary condition was fascistoid admiration, it would not follow that admiration of all sport stars is fascistoid.

Among 'physical characteristics crucial to success in sport' that in the nearer future may be possible to genetically design Tännsjö lists 'the capacity for oxygen uptake' and 'muscular volume' (p. 60). But these characteristics are not crucial to success in many sports. Let us make a rough distinction between two kinds of sports that I will call record sports and game sports. In record sports, you measure a certain capacity: you measure how fast competitors can run, ski, cycle, swin, etc. a certain distance, how high or long they can jump, how much they can lift, how far they can throw certain objects, and so on. In these sports, you may compete against yourself, trying to break your own record as well as interpersonal records. In game sports, you play a game according to certain rules. An opponent is usually necessary, and often there are team mates with whom you co-operate. Billiards, tennis and football are examples of popular game sports.

Now to generalize in a way that admittedly allows exceptions, scoring high with respect to the above mentioned simple physical characteristics is much more important for success in record sports than in game sports. For instance, great capacity for oxygen uptake is more important in being a good long-distance runner, cross-country skier or cyclist, and muscle volume is more important in being a good weight-lifter, wrestler or American Football player than any such characteristics are for being a good golfer or table-tennis player, let alone billiard player. So, even if we could genetically design people with a great capacity for oxygen uptake or with a disposition to develop a massive muscle volume, we would not be able to design people who are guaranteed to succeed in game sports.

Since some game sports are also team sports, like football, there is also the further difficulty that, even if you could genetically design footballers who are individually outstanding, it is quite a different matter to get them to play together successfully in a team. For such reasons, I do not think that any advances in the biological sciences are likely to have any marked influence on game sports in the foreseeable future.

What about record sports? Even here I think the impact of future biological discoveries will be far less extensive than Tännsjö imagines. The reason is that, apart from being blessed with advantageous physical assets of the sort mentioned, becoming a star in record sports takes at least having the right mental attitude, the dedication to a sport required to go through years of hard training. Thus, unless we look forward to a time when we can genetically design the right mindset or attitude for a sport – and at that time we will probably be able to genetically design prominent artists and scientists as well – all biological scientists could presumably do is to pick out youths with the required sports interest and work on them to improve their physique. But then the room for improving the capacity for oxygen uptake and so on will be severely restricted as compared to what it would be if scientists could work upon embryos. Perhaps not much more could be achieved than could by achieved by a refinement of the kinds of drugs now in use. So, contrary to what Tännsjö suggests, the situation is not at all similar to the one that obtains in the Formula 1 circuit (p. 64): we do not have the same potential to design powerful bodies in youths with the right mental attitude as we have to construct powerful cars for competent drivers.

A REFUTATION OF DESERT

Even if what we admire in sport stars, as well as in other people, are certain performances, and the efforts they have intentionally made are a necessary condition for this, it does not follow that admiration is justified. For there is a metaphysical argument to the effect that, ultimately, we are not responsible for any of the features we have.[5] Let us put this as an argument against desert, since it is in virtue of involving this notion that the argument tells against admiration (and contempt, pride, shame, etc.).

We have seen that desert is a consideration of justice:

> (1) If you deserve reward or punishment in virtue of having a feature F, it is just that you are rewarded or punished because you have F.

This requires that there be a certain proportion between the value of your having F and the value of the return you deserve. For instance, if you have made sacrifices to do good to others, the reward you deserve, or what it is just that you receive, in virtue of this fact is proportionate to the sacrifices you have endured and the good you have done. Similarly, for the punishment you deserve if you have prospered because of the harm you have done to others.

We have also seen:

> (2) It can be just to reward or punish you for having F only if you are responsible for having F.

For instance, it would not be just to punish some infants because they cause their mothers a lot of pain when they are born, and reward other infants who cause their mothers little pain because these infants are not responsible for the amount of pain they cause their mothers when they are born.

Now, when you are responsible for having F, you are so in virtue of having certain properties – call them 'responsibility-giving features'. These features do not include every feature that is causally necessary for your being responsible for having F, through being necessary for your very existence – e.g., such general conditions as the occurrence of the Big Bang or the presence of oxygen – but only features causally necessary and sufficient to determine whether, given your existence, the properties you possess include the particular property of being responsible for having F.

If you are responsible for having F, this is likely to be something that you have intentionally brought about. But to intentionally bring about that you have F, you must have certain information about the situation you are in, a character which inclines you to intend to bring about that you have F and abilities that allow you to execute this intention, and so on. It is possible that you are responsible for your having these particular responsibility-giving features, G. But if so, this must be in virtue of having certain other responsibility-giving features, H, which make you responsible for your having G. Evidently, this regress of responsibility cannot be infinite. Instead:

> (3) If you are responsible for your having F, this must ultimately be in virtue of responsibility-giving properties that you are not responsible for having.

In other words, even if you are responsible for having F, you are not ultimately reponsible for it. Now:

(4) It cannot be just to reward or punish you on the basis of your having these ultimate responsibility-giving properties.

Surely, this can be just as little as it can be just to punish and reward infants in accordance with whether they cause their mothers much or little pain when born. In both cases, the explanations of the properties refer to natural forces beyond the subject's responsibility.

However:

(5) If it cannot be just to reward or punish you on the basis of those of your properties which ultimately account for your being (directly) responsible for having F, it cannot be just to reward or punish you on the basis of your having F.

For this is indirectly to reward or punish you on the basis of the ultimate responsibility-giving properties on the basis of which it is agreed that it cannot be just to reward and punish you. It cannot be just to reward or punish you, and thereby make you better or worse off than others, on the basis of properties you are guaranteed to have by properties you are not responsible for having and others are prevented from having through lacking properties beyond their responsibility.

An analogy between responsibility and justification may help to clarify this argument. Suppose you justify your belief that p in terms of your belief that q. The latter belief in its turn is justfied in terms of the belief that r. Arguably, this regress cannot be infinite. So, imagine r is left without justification. Then, although p is justified in terms of q which in its turn is justified by r, there is ultimately no justification for p. Similarly, if you are described as being responsible for your having F in virtue of having responsibility-giving features, G, for which you are responsible in virtue of having H, for which you are not responsible. Although you are – directly – responsible for having F, even in virtue of having properties for which you are in turn (directly) responsible, you are not ultimately responsible for having F.

Direct responsibility is sufficient for a forward-looking justification of the practice of reward and punishment, in terms of the beneficial consequences of this practice for you and other agents. For if you are directly responsible for your actions in virtue of acting on the basis of certain intentions you have, rewards and punishments can change your future behaviour by making you form different intentions in the future. However, saying that to reward and punish you on the basis of your having F is deserved is saying that there is a backward-looking justification which requires ultimate responsibility, a proportion between the value of this return and something for which you are ultimately responsible that makes the return just. But we cannot be ultimately responsible for anything. Ultimately, the explanation of our responsibility-giving properties will be in terms of features for which we cannot be responsible. To reward and punish on the basis of properties for which we are not ultimately responsible is as little just as it is to reward and punish babies for causing their mothers little or much pain when born.

To sum up. The practice of rewarding and punishing on the basis of our having F (e.g., our having done a certain action) can be deserved and just only if we are responsible for having F. But since we are always responsible for something, such as having F, in virtue of having some other properties, G (e.g., forming a certain intention), the question arises why we have G. If we are not responsible for having G, it seems that it cannot after all be more just to reward or punish us on the basis of F than it would be if we were not (directly) responsible for having F. For indirectly this is to reward or punish us on the ground of properties for which we are not responsible, properties which guarantee that we will be responsible for F and exclude those who lack them from this responsibility. But eventually, since we are temporally finite beings, we are bound to arrive at responsibility-giving properties for which we are not responsible; the regress of responsibility cannot be infinite. So, we cannot possess the ultimate responsibility which is requisite to make rewarding and punishing deserved and just. Only the forward-looking mode of justification, which yields only direct responsibility, can be vindicated.

By refuting the applicability of the concept of desert, this argument makes rationally unjustifiable all emotions that involve this concept, such as admiration, contempt, pride and shame. The argument does not rule out, however, our positive or negative evaluations of human performances and, thus, not emotions such as liking (approval, love, etc.) and dislike (disapproval, hatred, etc.) of human beings. It does, however, show that were these evaluations to lead us to create a world in which some are better off than others – as they would in the hands of fascists – this would be unjust and, thus, if they cannot be morally justified in any other way, wrong. Thus, this argument explains what could be morally wrong with fascistoid attitudes as they have here been construed.

CONCLUSION

As opposed to Tännsjö, I have argued that we ought not welcome genetic engineering in sport because it will make our admiration of sport stars disappear, which would be a good thing because this admiration, being based on strength, is fascistoid. First, admiration of strength cannot be shown to be fascistoid by being linked to a contempt for weakness in the way Tännsjö imagines. Second, although an admiration of somebody because of a property outwith their responsibility is unjustifiable, it is not what makes it fascistoid. Although they do not involve erroneous attributions of responsibility, attraction and repulsion can be fascistoid if they block out concern for well-being. Hence, by placing strength within our responsibility, genetic engineering would allow fascistoid tendencies to express themselves in the emotion of admiration. Third, it is only in some sports that having physical strength or some other simple physical power to a higher degree than normal is even a necessary condition for an admirable performance. Therefore, genetic manipulation of these physical factors would have little effect upon our admiration of sport stars. Fourth, there is, however, a metaphysical argument that displays the injustice of admiration and other desert-involving emotions, irrespective of whether their objects are sport stars or other human beings. This argument shows what is wrong or immoral about fasciostoid attitudes: they involve the injustice of treating some worse than others on the basis of some properties that do not make this just or morally justified in any other way.

NOTES

1   Chapter 5 in this volume.
2   It might be objected that we speak of such a thing as *self*-contempt. This is possible, I conjecture, when we regard ourselves as so inferior that we are alienated from ourselves and, thus, no longer feel shame. Significantly, there is no such thing as self-admiration for when we approve of ourselves we are not alienated from ourselves. There is here room for nothing but pride.
3   Claudio Tamburrini makes a similar point in a critique of an earlier paper by Tännsjö. See Tamburrini's 'Sports, Fascism, and the Market', *Journal of the Philosophy of Sport*, 25, 1998: 35–47, 42–3.
4   This point is obscured when Tännsjö writes: 'Some people tend to admire the great scientist or the outstanding artist, not their accomplishments' (p. 00). The truth is that people admire these people *because* of their accomplishments, which they find valuable in one way or another.
5   An argument analogous to the one I am about to set forth has been formulated by Galen Strawson: 'The Impossibility of Moral Responsibility', reprinted in Louis P. Pojman and Owen McLeod, *What Do We Deserve?* (New York: Oxford University Press, 1999).

7 Educational or genetic blueprints, what's the difference?

Claudio Tamburrini

INTRODUCTION

Following the use of genetic technology to prevent and cure different pathological conditions, we may face the possibility of enhancing athletic performances through genetic engineering in a not-so-far-ahead future. In theory, genetic interventions could be effected either on an already existing person (somatic genetic modifications) or at an embryo level (germ-line genetic modifications), in order to improve certain physiological characteristics that enhance athletic performance (for instance, the capacity for oxygen uptake or the propensity for muscular growth).[1] In the case of germ-line modifications, the transformed genetic structure will be inherited by the modified person's offspring.

Most people, including those who believe gene technology could be made relatively safe from a medical point of view in the future, see the eventual arrival of this new technique as a fundamental threat to sports and society. Regarding sports, these people believe gene doping subverts the ideal of fair competition, that is not only central to sports, but even has educational value for the new generations.

In this chapter, I will discuss an objection to gene doping based on the ideal of personal autonomy. As Ivo van Hilvoorde rightly points out in this volume (Chapter 8), gene technology provides a new, dramatic dimension to the 'educational paradox' – as formulated by Kant in his question 'How do I cultivate freedom through coercion?' Focusing mainly on germ-line genetic modifications, I will question whether the 'genetic design' of a (still unborn) child is a fundamental threat to, or even a denial of, that child's personal autonomy. And I will also ask whether genetic pre-programming essentially differs from the stimulation and specialisation considered to be legitimate aims of good education and upbringing.

Throughout my discussion, I will distinguish two different ways in which a person's autonomy might be violated, and will then argue that genetic technology does not violate either of them. As a corollary to this discussion, a notion of autonomy better adapted to the challenge posed by the new emerging genetic technologies will be sketched which recommends, rather than banishes, germ-line modifications of our offspring. Finally, I will also try to substantiate the claim that the ban on gene doping runs counter to individuals' right to privacy and to fundamental notions of legal security, and should therefore be abolished.

GENE TECHNOLOGY REDUCES INDIVIDUALS' RANGE OF ACTION

Let me first dispose of one objection to the application of genetic technology, either in sports or in education in general, that will not hit the mark. The objection runs as follows: as the new technology is dangerous, both on a somatic or an embryonic level, it threatens to seriously impair individuals' autonomy. According to a notion of autonomy, individuals are autonomous when they are able to entertain different courses of actions without impediments. Thus, a person could be more or less autonomous, depending on the number and degree of activities he or she is able to undertake. The more reduced my range of action is, the less autonomous I am. Suffering from a serious handicap, as the ones a gene-modified person may be affected by if the intervention goes wrong, reduces the number of options open to that person, thereby diminishing their autonomy.

Although laudable in its intention, the present objection does not hold all the way. At present, not even sceptics doubt that new genetic technologies have the potential to prevent and cure serious diseases. This insight explains the acceptance this particular application of genetic technology enjoys, both at a social and at a legal level. That means that, unlike traditional doping techniques, genetic technology will be widely used (as a matter of fact, it is already being used) in general medicine. Before the new techniques are introduced in other areas of society, for instance, sports medicine and education, they will first be developed and tested in the health care system. Even if genetic modification today still involves some risks, it will most probably be as harmless as a medical technique can be in the future, following its medical applications.[2] At least, no more harmful than current elite training techniques. Thus, genetically modified individuals will not be exposed to any morally relevant risks. No relevant impairment of personal autonomy occurs therefore with this new form of 'doping', in the sense discussed above. And as many people today oppose traditional doping mainly on the grounds that it is dangerous for athletes, opponents of gene doping will then be deprived of their main argument for the ban.

GENE TECHNOLOGY DEPRIVES INDIVIDUALS OF CONTROL OVER THEIR LIVES

According to a second notion of autonomy, a person is autonomous in relation to the degree to which he or she can decide on their life projects, goals and plans. Thus, a person can be said to be (more or less) autonomous, depending on the level of control he or she has over important matters in his or her life. Accordingly, it is said, genetic interventions at the embryonic level violates individuals' autonomy, as modified persons are designed to fit certain activities before they are even born. Or so objectors to gene technology could argue for their cause.

What could be said about this argument? There is no doubt that the new techniques carry with them a threat to personal autonomy, in the sense of introducing (still) a risky, manipulative factor in the pedagogical process. But, in that regard, gene technologies do not essentially differ from traditional education. Also a bad educator may turn out to reduce the educand's control over his or her life options. A mere 'threat' to personal autonomy cannot therefore justify a ban on genetic modification. Widely stated, any decision taken by parents or educators constitutes a possible threat to the child's autonomy.

Rather, the question is whether gene technology implies a fundamental denial of individual autonomy. What does such a denial amount to? Roughly, this could mean that there are no other ways of life the educand could freely choose from, besides the one imposed by the pedagogic programme. A blueprint is thus 'executed' without leaving any alternatives open for the child and, often, not even for the parents. The absence of a critical attitude regarding the pre-existing blueprint hampers any educational adaptation to the specific character and wishes of the child (as can be the case when children are made to compete in elite sport contexts).

More precisely, the present objection states that the educand is denied an autonomous life project, in a fundamental way, when he or she is presented with given, external life goals, projects, etc., which are not of their own choosing because they have had no say in their formulation. Genetic pre-programming an individual to excel in a particular activity constitutes, objectors would say, an example of 'targeted' pedagogy and is therefore a powerful denial of that person's autonomy. We should abstain from using that technique, and leave instead the decision on whether or not to undertake a particular path in life to the individual him or herself.

To begin with, as formulated, this objection is too comprehensive. It affects not only gene technology, but also the sort of specialisation in a certain activity – and the predisposition for it so generated – that characterise traditional education. Both parents and teachers inculcate daily certain skills and attitudes in our children that will certainly influence their professional choices. Why do we see this kind of 'pre-programming' as less objectionable than genetic engineering?

For many people, the answer is obvious. A good education instills in the child a variety of skills, giving the child the necessary self-confidence to make free, autonomous decisions. Far from pre-programming or predisposing the child to adopt a particular path in life, the good pedagogue allows the educand's personality to flourish and, when the time comes, to freely choose the abilities he or she wants to reassert by following a particular professional career. To put it succinctly: traditional education widens the educand's horizons, while genetic technology makes it narrower.

I cannot see why genetic technology would be incompatible with this pedagogic ideal. It is true that, unlike what happens in traditional education, the genetically modified child would know from the very beginning that, if he or she so chooses, they can be really good at, say, field and track disciplines or mathematics. But this does not compel him or her to become a sportsman/sportswoman or a mathematician, any more than the good teacher 'compels' a child to become a lawyer when he reasserts the child's ability for legal issues. It seems exaggerated to affirm that genetic technology narrows the educand's range of life plans and projects. On the contrary, if knowledge yields power to influence one's own life, genetically transformed educands will be more empowered than traditional students.

But is it not problematic enough to know in advance what one is good at? Such information might, for instance, cause anxiety in some children and risk influencing their future professional choices too much. Compare this situation with genetic counselling and the information given to individuals regarding their susceptibility to generate specific kinds of disease. There is a possibility that the psychological trauma invoked by such knowledge is more detrimental than the disease itself. (Some people go so far as to suggest that this knowledge might even provoke the onset of the disease in question.)

However, in my view, such a comparison is misleading. Knowing in advance about your skills and abilities cannot reasonably be compared with being informed about what diseases you might develop in the future. In the context of a proper pedagogical environment, the first kind of information is 'good news'. It cannot therefore be expected to provoke the same traumatic effect as knowing about the predisposition for a serious disease can have.

In that regard, genetic technology is no more problematic than vocational testing. Vocational tests also tell the child in advance what he or she could do well at. Should we then forbid these tests too? Many adolescents might even feel relieved to know that, if they so wish, there is a professional area in which they can excel. Genetic technology, as a more sophisticated form of vocational testing, can give them that, at least as a non-intended side-effect.

GENE TECHNOLOGY ENHANCES INDIVIDUAL AUTONOMY

If my arguments in the section above are right, it cannot be concluded that genetically designing a person to fit a particular social or professional activity before he or she is even born amounts to a violation of that individual's autonomy. However, this conclusion is a rather defensive one. I believe a more affirmative stance can be substantiated on the basis of the preceding arguments. It could be stated as follows: If a person can be said to be (more or less) autonomous, depending on the level of control he or she has on important matters of their life, then that person has a right to be genetically modified, provided such engineering is conducive to a broader dominion of life options in the future.

Suppose I am offered the possibility of neutralising a gene in my offspring that affects muscle elasticity at a certain age. By means of genetic engineering, my child will then get rid of muscle tissue decay until much later in life than most other people. On which ethical grounds can this futuristic right to modification supposedly owed to people still unborn be justified?

Provided the improvement to my child's life quality is substantial, and given it is possible to perform the gene-surgical intervention with a reasonable level of risk, a consequentialist approach to ethics would recommend such action as welfare-maximising, other things being equal. According to the most widespread version of consequentialist ethics, we should maximise the welfare, not only of those people who actually will exist in the future, but also of possible people.[3] From this follows a duty to bring about the existence of as many people as possible, who can be expected to live a life that is worth living. There are good reasons not to limit this reasoning to people. Something similar might, for instance, be argued regarding skills and traits. If some physical or psychological character-istic can reasonably be expected to enhance its bearer's quality of life, without negatively affecting other (actual, future or possible) people, then we are under a consequentialist duty to actualise that trait.

Of course, to this it could be argued that such a defence of the genetic engineering of future generations rests on a very narrow, and strongly questioned, ethical approach. After all, it could be said, not everyone is a consequentialist, even less a total, impersonal utilitarian.

Would, for instance, a right-based ethical approach come to a different con-clusion regarding the example above? Let us recall that it is not the case that, as a consequence of the genetic intervention, my child will be deprived of life options. Genetic programming, like sound education, predisposes but does not determine. So, we would definitely not be depriving my offspring of the possibility of choosing for herself who to become and which path of life to follow. As a matter of fact, according to the first notion of autonomy discussed above, my child might even be said to have a right to be born as well equipped and prepared as possible, in order to confront the vicissitudes of life with a fair chance of success. If I don't manipulate her genome, she might as an adult accuse me of not giving her a good start in life (again, the parallel with education is obvious). So, rather than violating the right to self-determination of my offspring, I would be securing it by enlarging her skills and traits repertoire.

Finally, what would a virtue-based approach to ethics have to say about the prospect of enhancing my offspring genetically before birth? In my view, what is central to the variety of theories that could be included in this stream of thought is the emphasis put on developing one's potentialities, in order to make our human condition flourish. I see no reason to dismiss the possibility of accentuating this personality development process by other means than traditional education. At least, provided the two previously discussed ideals of personal autonomy are not transgressed.

THE BAN ON GENE DOPING AND INDIVIDUALS' RIGHT TO PRIVACY

There is another problematic aspect of the ban on genetic enhancements in sports. In order to check that athletes are abiding by the prohibition, it will be necessary to test them for genetic traits. This constitutes a violation of athletes' right to privacy. To begin with, the tests might reveal information they do not want, for instance, about their propensity to develop certain serious diseases. Second, this information might be misused by third parties, for instance, insurance companies and employers, against the athletes.

Here it could be argued that, if you want to be a part of the game, then you are required to abide by the rules imposed by sport organisations. I find this argument extremely bureaucratic and short-sighted. Let us recall that the IOC itself abolished sex testing before the Olympic Games at Sydney 2000 with the argument that such testing violated women athletes' integrity. It is true that, by the time it was abolished, sex testing has become discredited among women athletes and the public opinion. But I think the same could be said about genetic testing. Most of us feel, and rightly so, that revealing our genetic constitution is a threat to our privacy.[4] Besides, even if the World Antidoping Agency (WADA), the IOC and other international sport federations could manage to get 'acceptance' for the genetic testing from athletes, we should not forget that, by testing the athletes, the genetic constitution of their relatives will also be revealed. So, their families also will be given information on their genetic constitution they might not wish to have. And they might also be submitted to the risk of being discriminated by employers or insurance companies. To sum up: testing for gene doping violates not only the privacy of those submitted to the testing, it also exposes third parties to harm.

THE BAN ON GENE DOPING AND LEGAL SECURITY

Even if WADA, the IOC and other sport federations decide to ignore the objection above, there still is another problematic aspect of the ban that touches upon individuals' legal security. Let me return to my previous example of genetically manipulating my (still unborn) daughter. If I decide to go along with this procedure, she will be endowed with excellent physiological qualities that will give her considerable advantages in the exercise of a particular sport activity (that could be, for example, a higher than normal concentration of red blood cells). When the time comes for her to start competing, she is nonetheless denied the right to participate in sport competitions because of her irregular blood count (or, if first allowed, she will then be banned from further competition on grounds of being doped). Is it reasonable to punish her for something she didn't do?

In the 1960s, the Finnish cross-country skier Eero Mäntyranta was suspected of blood doping because his red blood count was 20 per cent higher than that of his competitors. Thirty years later, 200 members of his whole family were tested by scientists, and they found that fifty of them, including Mäntyranta himself, had been born with a rare genetic mutation that causes an increase in oxygen-rich red blood cells. This mutation gave Mäntyranta a competitive advantage in front of his rivals. Now, why would it have been wrong, or contrary to the ideal of fairness in competition, to give Mäntyranta's competitors the possibility of equalising competitive conditions by resorting to old-fashioned blood doping or, if it had been available at that time, to genetically caused EPO-doping? And what would the morally relevant difference be between my daughter's blood count and Mäntyranta's, that could justify banning her from competition, but not him?

Many people think artificial enhancing methods are obviously unacceptable, and tend to cling to the idea that only natural talent should decide the outcome of a sport competition. I find that idea difficult to substantiate. Why should congenital, genetically determined traits lead to victory and praise, but not acquired ones? Such a notion of justice is not only flawed, it is also becoming obsolete, due to the pace of medical development that is taking place today. There is no reason to let the genetic lottery decide a sport competition, when the winning odds of the competitors might be levelled out by intentional and goal-oriented efforts to achieve a higher sport performance level.

By resorting to the dubious distinction between 'natural' and 'artificial' qualities, one could at best ban my daughter from competition, but not her offspring. If one still wants to prohibit this kind of genetic enhancement, then it will be necessary to proscribe a whole family, included generations yet to come. Otherwise, if my daughter's offspring were allowed to participate on grounds that they were not responsible for their physiological characteristics, the ban on genetic enhancements would become invalid.

CONCLUSION

My conclusions are as follows:

1   Regarding the notion of autonomy that underlines reducing the range of actions open to an agent, developments in genetic technique probably will lead to relatively harmless genetic modifications, no more risky than the highly specialised elite training techniques used at present. No violation of personal autonomy occurs, in the sense discussed here.

2   Concerning the charge that genetic technology deprives the educand of control over his or her life by inculcating on them external, heteronomous reasons for action, I have admitted that genetic technology, and knowledge about the genetically designed educational programme, might no doubt predispose the educand to choose a particular professional career. But predisposition is not the same as determination. Besides, knowing in advance what one could be good at because of a genetic predisposition might neutralise much of the worry young people feel, caused by their not knowing what they are suited to in professional life.

3   Genetic engineering of the still unborn child might even be advocated as a consequentialist duty impending upon us, or alternatively as a right of our offspring to get as good as possible start in life. Thus, a positive ideal of personal autonomy could be formulated, according to which children of the future should not be deprived of the opportunity to be genetically modified.

4   Finally, regarding the ban by WADA and the ruling sport organisations on genetic doping, I have argued that the prohibition is not only unreasonable,

but even impossible to implement while paying due respect to current ideals of individuals' right to privacy and legal security.

NOTES

1 This use of genetic technology in sport medicine is nowadays popularly called 'gene doping'. Of course, somatic genetic modification may also be dangerous for an existing individual. Is this particularly disturbing for somatic gene modifications? I do not think so. The desirability of strengthening personal autonomy – itself a warrant against intrusive state intervention in individuals' private sphere – proposes allowing every individual to decide for themself which risks he or she is willing to take in order to achieve professional success and recognition, as long as this does not substantially affect others. However, I will not expand on this, as I have already discussed this subject in a previous work. For a more thorough discussion on this, see my article 'What's wrong with doping?', in T. Tännsjö, and C.M. Tamburrini, (eds) (2000) *Values in Sport: Elitism, Nationalism, Gender Equality and the Scientific Manufacture of Winners* (London: E & FN Spon), pp. 200–16.

2 The possibility of genetic engineering becoming rather safe in the future is, if not affirmatively asserted, at least not dismissed by Peter Schjerling in his contribution to this volume on p. 29.

3 This variant of consequentialism, usually known as total impersonal consequentialism, has some problems, for instance 'the repugnant conclusion', as formulated by Derek Parfit (see *Reasons and Persons*, Part 4, especially Chapter 17, pp. 381–90). However troublesome this objection might appear to be for total consequentialists, other authors (for instance, one of the co-editors of this volume) do not consider the repugnant conclusion as fatal for the theory. See, on this, T. Tännsjö, *Hedonistic Utilitarianism* (Edinburgh: Edinburgh University Press, 1998).

4 A survey supported financially by the EU Commission showed that a clear majority of those interviewed are opposed to authorities and insurance companies obtaining genetic information about individuals. In Sweden and Denmark, this opposition was as high as 93 per cent of the people consulted. In Spain, Portugal and Greece, 75 per cent of those interviewed were opposed to it, while other EU countries show figures somewhere in between.

REFERENCES

Munthe, Christian (1999) 'Genetic Treatment and Preselection: Ethical Differences and Similarities', in A. Nordgren (ed.) *Gene Therapy and Ethics*. Uppsala: Acta Universitatis Upsaliensis, pp. 159–72.

Munthe, Christian (2000) 'Selected Champions: Making Winners in the Age of Genetic Technology', in T. Tännsjö and C.M. Tamburrini (ed.), *Values in Sport, Elitism, Nationalism, Gender Equality and the Scientific Manufacture of Winners*. London: E & FN Spon, pp. 217–31.

Parfit, Derek (1988) *Reasons and Persons*, Oxford: Clarendon Press.

Tamburrini, Claudio (2000a) 'What's Wrong with Doping?', in T. Tännsjö and C. M. Tamburrini (eds) *Values in Sport: Elitism, Nationalism, Gender Equality and the Scientific Manufacture of Winners*. London: E & FN Spon, pp. 200–16.

Tamburrini, Claudio (2000b) *The 'Hand of God'?: Essays in the Philosophy of Sports*. Göteborg: Acta Universitatis Gothoburgensis.

Tännsjö, Torbjörn (1998) *Hedonistic Utilitarianism*, Edinburgh: Edinburgh University Press.

Tännsjö, Torbjörn (2000b) 'Is It Fascistoid to Admire Sports Heroes?", in T. Tännsjö and C.M. Tamburrini (eds) *Values in Sport*. London: E & FN Spon, pp. 9–23.

Tännsjö, Torbjörn and Tamburrini, Claudio (eds) (2000) *Values in Sport: Elitism, Nationalism, Gender Equality and the Scientific Manufacture of Winners*. London: E & FN Spon.

8 Sport and genetics

Moral and educational considerations regarding 'athletic predestination'

Ivo van Hilvoorde

INTRODUCTION

Recent biotechnological developments raise fundamental questions about the future of sports. Genetical research confronts both elite and recreational sports with its critical limits at the 'minimum' and the 'maximum' level of functioning. Several large research programs are searching for the location of crucial genes that are related to sport performance (cf. Montgomery *et al.*, 1998; Rankinen *et al.*, 2001; Wolfarth, 2002). Jason Gulbin, working with young talents for the Australian Sport Federation, says:

> Yes, it's a bit of a race . . . genes account for a lot between performances. So unlocking the answer to that is big business. . . . From our point of view it's worth looking at the fact that our population compared with, say the USA and China, is very small, and so I think we've got to be smarter about maximising the talent we have. . . . if we want to remain internationally competitive, we have to do things in a smart way. So the race to find out the performance enhancing genes is definitely on.[1]

Within the world of sports, the expectation is growing that in the near future the first genetically modified athlete will enter the sport arena. In 1997 Bouchard *et al.* suggested that in the very near future (within the next ten to fifteen years) genetic engineering of superelite athletes will not only be possible, but also routinely practiced in certain corners of the globe (Singer *et al.*, 1999: 146). 'Doping will become obsolete', according to Tamburrini, 'as it will be replaced by the genetic engineering of winners.' (2000: 153).

By now, various biogenetical scientists temper these high expectations, such as Bouchard himself: 'The human genome map has shown the situation is more complex than we believed. . . . Even clear targets, involving a single gene or small group of genes, may require another century of research' (in Miah, 2002: 180). Recently a special issue of the *Deutsche Zeitschrift für Sportmedizin* had some reservations on the topic: 'At the moment it is rather unlikely that in the near future the fiction of the genetically modified athlete will become reality' (Steinacker and Wolfarth, 2002).

But in spite of the reservation in their conclusions, these research programs reinforce the suggestion that, in the long run, sport-relevant features can be localized in our genes. And after localizing these genes, the next step of modification, using the knowledge for some kind of enhancement seems to be a small one. What are the consequences of these new techniques to enhance human performance? In this chapter I will discuss just a few of the many issues involved. I will respond to the position advanced by Tamburrini in this volume, where he defends the legitimate use of genetic enhancement within sports. The major questions I will address are how 'athletic predestination' of a child may threaten or deny personal autonomy and how genetic modification can influence the concept of 'equal opportunities' in sport.

My comments on the argument of Tamburrini will concentrate on three points of discussion. I will first focus on the concept of education. Does the analogy between genetic enhancement and education imply a limited – teleological – conception of education? The second point concerns the rather 'unempirical' character of Tamburrini's argument, that is the implicit premise that there are direct and equal opportunities for all in case of genetic enhancement. Third, I will comment on Tamburrini's argument concerning the mistaken polarity between enhancement, on the one hand, and dedication and character excellence, on the other. How does this polarity relate to a possible shift of admiration of sport heroes in the case of genetically designed athletes?

EDUCATION AS PRE-PROGRAMMING?

Does 'athletic predestination' of a child mean a fundamental denial of the personal autonomy of that child? 'Not necessarily', is Tamburrini's answer. He thereby makes an analogy between pre-programming and specialisation that can also be the aims of good education and upbringing (this volume, p. 84). According to Tamburrini, 'pre-programming' an individual does not need to run counter to the ideal of a good education nor to pedagogical ideals in giving guidance and support, developing a variety of skills and being attentive to the preferences and skills of the child. Tamburrini argues that gene technology carries a threat to personal autonomy, but does not imply a fundamental denial of individual autonomy.

Methods of education and stages of development cannot be understood without making clear what the developmental criteria are based on.[2] We can all agree on clear goals of education as well as fundamental rights, such as the right to an open future (Davis, 1997, 2001). However, what are the criteria on which we can judge our educational acts that run counter to these ideals? What about 'autonomy' as an educational goal? One can claim that any decision by parents or any coercive act means a possible threat to autonomy. This 'educational paradox' – as formulated by Kant in his question 'How do I cultivate freedom through coercion?' (1964: 711) – does not need to contradict autonomy as a leading principle of education and upbringing. Education is a process in which the personhood of the child is simultaneously affirmed and denied (Biesta, 1994). To say that the autonomy is fundamentally being denied means that there are clearly no alternative ways of life. A blueprint is 'executed' without alternatives for both parents and child. The absence of a critical attitude regarding the pre-existing blueprint limits any educational adaptation of the specific character and wishes of the child. Such a denial of autonomy can be defined as indoctrination, which means the deliberate attempt to still the development of a critical attitude (Spiecker and Straughan, 1991).

This can be illustrated by the difference between the 'natural born' son of Steffi Graf and Andre Agassi and an imaginary reproductive clone of John McEnroe. Both babies might be equally predestined to become elite tennis players. Although Graf and Agassi have eliminated a considerable amount of anthropological pre-game chance factors (cf. Breivik, 2000), when their child decides to become a tennis player too, it is still plausible that it will remain the choice of the child itself to play tennis, or not.[3] The wish to duplicate McEnroe because of his tennis talent is something else. Resistance to reproductive cloning (and genetic enhancement) with the aim of passing on a certain talent, is (besides matters of safety) primarily an objection against an instrumental relation with the offspring, the idea of exploiting talent and endangering the right to an open future.

I do not claim that genetic enhancement necessarily leads to indoctrination, nor that it precludes good education. I do, however, question the significance of the analogy between education and bioengineering. In the eyes of Tamburrini, pre-programming an individual to excel in the exercise of a sporting activity is not fundamentally different from the sort of specialization in a certain activity that characterizes the education of children. He writes: 'Both parents and teachers inculcate daily certain skills and attitudes in our children that will certainly influence their professional choices.' He then follows: 'Why do we see this kind of "pre-programming" as less objectionable than genetic engineering?' (this volume, p. 84). In my opinion, it is not meaningful to ask why it is 'less objectionable', because the analogy falls short in general.

The concept of education is fundamentally different from pre-programming, because it denies education as being a communicative process in which the results are unknown by definition. Building on central insights from pragmatism, Biesta (1995, 1997) argues that education should be understood in terms of the coordination of action. This brings to the fore the radical unpredictability of education. The 'content' of education cannot be thought of as something preceding pedagogical interaction. The concept of pre-programming wrongly presupposes a clear goal that is intrinsically linked to the means that lead to this goal. 'Pre-programming' genes concerns modifying conditions preceding education, but not education itself.

The results of genetic enhancement eventually depend on the environment in which talents can be nurtured. In other words, the goals of education have to permeate each 'educational act'. According to Dewey:

> the only way in which adults consciously control the kind of education which the immature get is by controlling the environment in which they act, and

> hence think and feel. We never educate directly, but indirectly by means of the environment.
>
> (1916, cited in Biesta, 1997: 315)

My point is that it is not the enhancing *per se* that seems to be morally problematic. Instead, moral attention needs to be directed to the aims that precede the wish to modify genes and the effects these motivations will have on daily educational practice. In other words, what is relevant is the intention of genetic enhancement and the educational consequences. The Flying Finn, the runner Paavo Nurmi, won seven gold medals in the Olympic Games in 1924 and 1928. There is a story about his style of upbringing. Nurmi stretched the feet of his infant son to condition him to become a runner. His wife disapproved of this stretching. It was not so much the stretching as such that was problematic or harmful, but the intention that his son was being conditioned to become an elite runner, like his father.

I agree with Tamburrini that there is a parallel between genetic modification and early selection within elite sport. However, that does not mean that this is in all cases a good practice that needs to be followed. There is much evidence by now on the potential damaging effects of high-performance sport for children (cf. Adirim and Cheng, 2003; Tofler *et al.*, 1996; Tymowski, 1999). If freedom of choice, health and independence are of a higher order than a sub-goal like enhancing athletic talents, why put the higher order at risk by restricting the spectrum of choice?

Tamburrini leaves open the possibility that a genetically modified child – even when modified with the purpose of a specific career – has a future as open as any other child does. He writes:

> It is true that, unlike what happens in traditional education, the genetically modified child would know from the very beginning that, if he or she so chooses, they can be really good at, say, field and track disciplines or mathematics. But this does not compel him or her to become a sportsman/ sportswoman or a mathematician, any more than the good teacher 'compels' a child to become a lawyer when he reasserts the child's ability for legal issues. . . . Many adolescents might even feel relieved to know that, if they so wish, there is a professional area in which they can excel.
>
> (this volume, pp. 84–5)

In my view, this underestimates the 'bioengineering power' as opposed to 'educational influences'. Educational influence of the parents can be 'undone' to a certain extent. People can 're-educate' themselves when it comes to changing preferences, for example, quit playing the violin and start playing soccer instead. According to Cooke, the kind of influence parents would have in choosing the genetic endowment of future generations is different in kind, first, because it is not so easily changed, and second, because it may effect how and what future generations want to change about themselves (2003: 39). One generation cannot know which genetic traits would be best for a future generation, because one does not know what the conditions will be when the child grows up. To deny this openness of the future may result in 'intergenerational imperialism'.

It needs to be stressed that the use of genetic technology does not necessarily run counter to a right to an open future. In some cases, it may even enhance individual autonomy. Education needs a balance of ideals (as imagined excellences) and realistic expectations (De Ruyter, 2003). More knowledge on genetic make-up may be helpful to prevent trying to achieve athletic performance beyond the perceived capacities. Knowledge of genes may thus contribute to enhance human autonomy or even to the prevention of harm. 'Knowing thy – genetic – self' might help children to evaluate their capacities and to gain insight into the ideals that may be achievable. One can also imagine that potential grief will be spared for the non-selected since they will not frustrate the high ambitions of their parents. Children have a right to an honest insight into the feasibility of the high ambitions of their parents who are willing to offer their time and money with the prospect of sport success. The interests and autonomy of the child can be more carefully weighed against those of parents and coaches.

Biotechnology does run counter to the right to an open future when the freedom to bioengineer the offspring results in communities of people who share a common genetic structure and at the same time are alienated from other communities. 'Genetic communitarianism' might result in different communities coming to view their differences as no longer the result merely of commitment and persuasion, but of their different "'natures", with the result that these differences come to be regarded as irreconcilable.' (Buchanan *et al.*, 2000: 178).

Each life is limited by and directed through education, working environment and socio-economic status of parents. Systems of education also stimulate competition and separation of communities. However, there is a difference between education and genetic modification in terms of the experience (not essence) of differences in human 'nature'. The creation of different communities based on different natures stimulates the competition in enhancement techniques. The majority of people may be forced to internalise disproportionate social pressure as a result of the tyranny of a minority who choose to genetically enhance their offspring (see Wijsbek, 2000). Seeking competitive advantage through enhancements can be collectively self-defeating and thus harmful for everyone. Also, allowing a market to determine who may pursue competitive advantage will be unfair to those who lack financial means (Buchanan *et al.*, 2000: 181).

I agree with Cooke (2003: 35) that we should not turn our back to potentially good applications of genetic engineering, due to fears of the worst case scenario. That means that we have to distinguish two important questions: what kinds of enhancement bring about general capabilities and what kinds of enhancements interfere or infringe on the freedom of future generations (ibid.: 51)? Do we enhance genes with a general or with a specific purpose? 'General-purpose means' like sight or hearing are useful and valuable in carrying out nearly any plan of life or set of aims that humans typically have (cf. Buchanan *et al.*, 2000). These enhancements may contribute to major educational values such as autonomy, independence, responsibility, emancipation and rationality. The personal auton-omy of a child may be denied or threatened when enhancements are so specific that they are aimed at a specific career or a specific talent rather than a contribu-tion to general educational values. Methods which attempt to impose fixed attitudes and beliefs upon individuals (for example, the life of an elite athlete is the best there is) and which fail to promote their capacity for independent judgment are anti-educational (Campbell, 1990). 'Pre-programming' a child just aiming at 'athletic predestination' is irreconcilable with autonomy as an educational goal and threatens the right to an open future.

GENETIC ENHANCEMENT: EQUAL AND DIRECT OPPORTUNITIES FOR ALL?

Equality of opportunities is an important principle of modern education. Differ-entiation in the school system is based on differences in talent. Notwithstanding these differences of capacities, the ideal of equality remains in terms of using, developing and stimulating specific talents. Whether genetic technology fosters equal opportunities or not is at least uncertain. However, arguments in favor of genetic enhancement cannot ignore the possibility that initially only a small part of the population will profit from applications of biotechnology. Given the high costs of these possible applications the inequality of opportunities seems to be more explicitly linked to socio-economic status than is the case with most educational systems.

This argument does not apply when the opportunities are in fact equal for all. But this seems a more abstract ideal than the current ideal of equal opportunities in education. Using genetic technology with the aim of enhancing human capacities can never begin safely at one specific moment for all. That means that there will be large differences between the potential profits and losses. This temporal dimension cannot be ignored in the argumentation in favor of any new technology.

The genetic lottery results in large inequalities on many different scales. If genetic enhancement is to be an available and safe technique for all, how will this influence the equality or differences between people? Tamburrini does not reckon with the possibility that inequalities may increase; he even expects an equalizing effect among individuals. In a previous article, he states: 'Genetic technology makes it possible to reduce current gaps in skills and inherited traits between individuals' (2002: 261). But on what evidence is this suggestion based? Genetic modification may just as well accentuate some of the inequalities. Following a simple Dutch saying: a donkey will never turn into a racehorse.

What about equal opportunities in sport? When it is possible to modify human genes with the aim of enhancing athletic performance, are we then still measuring the relevant inequalities? The construction of equal opportunities in sport is not inconsistent with the certainty of unequal outcome. Sport always combines elements of control (mastered by means of certain skills) and elements of chance (not to be confused with uncertainty of the outcome). In the discussion on the balance between control and chance, it is important to distinguish between pre-game and in-game factors (Breivik, 2000: 149–51). Sport generally excludes as many 'in-game' chance factors as possible. Breivik pleads for the flourishing of chance during the pre-game period, including genetic make-up as a variant of 'anthropological chance'. All elements of chance that are relevant for winning a game should, in his view, be eliminated as far as possible. The primary distributive norm in sport should be meritocratic (Loland, 2002). A competition is supposed to proceed according to the postulate of formal equality and openness of the results (Bette and Schimank, 2001: 55).

If it is possible to genetically modify certain features, and thus to exclude elements of pre-game chance, it only has an equalising effect when Tamburrini is right that genetic technology makes it possible to reduce gaps in talents. But again, apart from the question whether gene technology leaves the necessary skills untouched, there is no reason to believe that gaps will be reduced instead of widened. Besides, given the high costs, it seems more realistic that initially only a small number of elite athletes will profit from biotechnological applications. Breivik's plea for a flourishing of anthropological chance during the pre-game period must therefore also be related to the (im)possibilities of watching over these norms. If some people do start to control these elements of genetic change, it forces the other competitors to make a choice. And that means that athletes who choose the 'flourishing' of anthropological chance in fact 'choose' no longer to be elite, with no gain whatsoever attached to this choice. In that sense, Tamburrini's suggestion that the choice to be weaker, less intelligent or uglier than average 'might yield respect for the individual who so chooses' (2002: 262) seems to me unempirical. On any scale of normality, not many parents will choose deliberately for 'less than average' for their own child. Take the possibility of enhancing the memory of a child. Soderberg (1998) addresses the question whether genetic enhancement of the average memory of a child should be considered a practice along the lines of orthodontics, music lessons and soccer leagues. Moral liberalism treats genetic enhancement as an extension of other ways that parents have to give their children special advantages. This could lead to a tyranny of the minority that tries to gain advantages for their children. It also raises the problem of future lawsuits against parents who failed to give their children the best possible genes.[4] The point made by Soderberg is that if we agree to allow parents to seek enhancement of a child's average memory, it ultimately reinforces the notion of an ideal or perfect type.

Tamburrini responds to this claim that the supposed tyranny of the normal or the tyranny of the perfect underestimates the strength of new trends and the changeable character of aesthetic and life ideals. But even when new trends and life ideals become more and more changeable, the 'weak', 'unintelligent' and 'ugly' will not profit in any way from this, other than that they might move to the more average range of normality. It is not realistic to think that someone would choose to be less than average, unless it is based on moral superiority (a capacity that might also be modifiable within this artificial portrayal of man). Also, the magnitude of differences between people does not necessarily correlate with the moral or public judgement of these differences. In other words, even small margins can lead to large differences in judgement, as is the case in elite sport. The so-called 'problem of the relative ends' ('for tall men to exist there must be short men'; 'It's not enough to succeed, others must fail') is based on a concept of normality with regard to a successful life. This concept is not as changeable as the concept of a lifestyle seems to suggest. Genes for a successful life cannot be switched off or on like a high-fashion item.

ENHANCEMENT, DEDICATION AND A SHIFT OF ADMIRATION

Sport is about measuring performances with the aim of comparing differences in talent and dedication. Competitive sports can be characterized as a rule-governed social practice in which the organization of equal opportunities (by way of constitutive rules and levels of performance) makes it possible to express relevant differences in abilities (Breivik, 2000; Steenbergen *et al.*, 2001; Loland, 2002). Cultural admiration of elite athletes may be directed to both talent and dedication. To be competitive within modern elite sports takes both talent and dedication in vast quantities. This will not change with genetic technology. Some arguments against the use of genetic modification are based on the false assumption that efforts and dedication will no longer be of importance. Biotechnology in sport cannot replace training effort. Instead of genetic enhancement replacing dedication, 'artificial' enhancement at the same time enhances 'human' dedication. 'Going through a technical procedure in order to acquire this gene involves much more of a struggle than being luckily equipped with the same gene from birth' (Munthe, 2002: 297).

Public admiration of athletes is related to expectations about 'natural performance'. Enhancing genes seems to violate ideas of the natural and what defines our unique and individual make-up. Although sport organizations are very interested in adhering to demarcations such as that between natural and artificial, or between a 'triumph of character' and a 'triumph of chemistry' (Wadler, 1999), this idea is based upon a vague polarity between the 'nature of the body' and 'unnatural constructs of culture' (Gugutzer, 2001; van Hilvoorde, 2003). Polarities between nature and culture do, however, influence the mediated images of athletes and through that the admiration of the public. Both public and sport organizations need contrasts. They need good and bad, admiration and condemnation, both Carl Lewis and Ben Johnson. Following on from dichotomies like these is a rather arbitrary moral distinction between the enhancement of genes and enhancement of the environment. The medical and elite sport environment that stimulates the practice of genetic enhancement is itself an industry of enhancement.

One argument against genetic enhancement is based on the idea that the admiration of athletes will no longer concentrate on physiological predisposition. Tamburrini is right in saying that admiration of athletes will continue to be concentrated on the sacrifices endured to actualize their genetic predisposition. But that is not the only thing. Especially within sports that are characterized by complex motor skills, admiration will also be directed to talented players who make us believe that it takes little effort to perform. Even the player who puts his talent at risk (George Best, for example) is the subject of admiration and heroism.

When certain features such as muscle force can be chosen, attention might also shift to other characteristics to be admired, including moral qualities of the athlete, the extent of identification and the role as a model. The child of Marion Jones and Tim Montgomery will probably be blessed with 'fast genes'. Of course, the public admiration will not exclusively be directed to genetic make-up but rather to how this child deals with the pressure of 'athletic predestination' and the pressure of dealing with a life in the shadow of two champions as parents.

The public might become more concentrated on 'normality' in an 'abnormal arena'. Emotional identification and accessibility are already two of the anchors for appreciation of sport journalists and fans. This fact can hardly be ignored from a commercial point of view. If the organic relation between elite and youth sport is lost and with that a realistic example or role model, admiration could turn into amazement, as we experience in the circus. Think, for example, of the concept of a beautiful body as is practiced in modern bodybuilding. Many people are rather filled with horror or pity when they see the – in their eyes – aberrations of body concepts. The generally accepted notions of beauty and gender strongly influence and limit admiration based on dedication. When a female athlete does not conform to dominant notions of femininity, when she evokes 'fears of the monstrous feminine' (Magdalinski and Brooks, 2002), it does not matter how hard she has worked to reach her goals, public admiration will be limited. Engineering a different class of people might result in a loss of common ground of valuing. In case of athletic endeavor, this means that the role of the public and the threat of alienation cannot be ignored in the argument over 'athletic predestination'.

CONCLUSION

In this chapter I have questioned the conceptual link between genetic modification of a child and education. Education is a process in which the rationality of the child is both affirmed and denied. It is a communicative process with an uncertain outcome. That means that an instrumental rationality between stimulation by the educator and specialization of the child is problematic. Specialization cannot be the goal of education itself. To enhance one specific feature by means of genetic modification seems a short-cut with an uncertain outcome. Of course, genetic engineering can improve the statistical expectations of the outcomes (Gardner, 1995). However, the suggestion that genetic enhancement relates to education is based on a false connection between genes and behaviour.

Making one preferred outcome dominant can lead to indoctrination, suppressing a critical disposition, inculcating belief without rational justification (Siegel, 1991: 34) and narrowing life to a guarded community. Genetic enhancement with a specific purpose inculcates the belief that one specific talent should be valued over other valuable things in life. It ignores other possible talents, health risks and openness to other options and communities. In the case of elite sports, it also ignores what Brown (1990) calls the 'Prudential Athletic Life'. That means two things:

1   'Requirements of equal concern'; our well-being when we are old is just as important as our well-being when we are young.
2   'Keeping options open'; a prudential outlook requires us to keep in mind that in the later stages of our lives we may well have different projects, different allegiances, and different priorities and values, and we will then also need to call on our abilities and resources to satisfy the demands of these stages. In our prudential reflections we must be able to abstract from our present concerns and allow for later passions.

I conclude with two examples that illustrate the potential conflict between the nurturing of sport talent and the prudential athletic life. The first example is a sport manager working in a school for sport talents. He is complaining about parents who derive status from the talents of their children. I quote this sport manager: 'Parents are scary. If children are becoming successful you should actually declare them orphans regulated by law.'[5] He pleads for a state system, in which talents can be nurtured.

Another example is a very talented Dutch woman tennis player, fifth on the world junior ranking, who stopped playing tennis recently because she was not enjoying the game any more. She became aware of the discrepancy between her direct environment that told her that she had a wonderful life and her own experience of that life. One of the coaches of the Tennis Association commented as follows on her decision: 'I think it is sad that a seventeen-year-old girl already decides to quit playing tennis. I'm afraid that she will regret this decision.'[6] The term 'already' is striking. In this context it is rational to make the choice for a 5-year-old girl to start focusing on a professional career. However, her sign of autonomy when she is 17, her act to decide for another way of life, is interpreted as irrational.

Both examples illustrate a rationality of suppressing autonomy. The choice of another way of life is a difficult decision because of the strong pressure of the environment. In a context where parents and coaches will even attempt to modify genes, it is not hard to imagine that there would be even more coercion involved. With the modification of genes, the environment also hands the belief to the child that these genes should be used for the specific career that is aimed for. You can tell a child when he or she is old enough to understand: 'You have the genes to become an outstanding athlete, but of course it is up to you to become a musician too, or whatever you want.' However, in such an 'enhanced environment' in which genetic modification seems a logical step, parents or coaches do not wait until the child is old enough to decide on their own. The choice 'against' one's 'own' talented genes seems irrational, because it is a choice against a totally 'enhanced environment'.

NOTES

1 Radio National, Sporty Science, with Amanda Smith (16 August 2002). Hypertext document: http://www.abc.net.au/rn/talks/8.30/sportsf/stories/s649467.htm.
2 The internal differentiation of scientific disciplines, in particular, the historical division between educational science and developmental psychology, has prevented a more integrated study of educational goals and means (see van Hilvoorde, 2002).
3 John McEnroe wants to forbid Jaden Gil (the son of Agassi and Graf) to play tennis, because it will be unfair on his opponents (http://www.spiegel.de/sport/).
4 A recent 'wrongful life claim' in the Netherlands – a child won a court case because she 'should not have been born' – illustrates that this is not merely speculation.
5 *Volkskrant*, 26 April 2003.
6 *Volkskrant*, 18 April 2003.

REFERENCES

Adirim, T.A. and Cheng, T.L. (2003) 'Overview of Injuries in the Young Athlete', *Sports Medicine*, 33(1): 75–81.

Andersen, J.L., Schjerling, P. & Saltin, B. (2000) 'Muscle, Genes and Athletic Performance', *Scientific American*, 283: 30–7.

Aschwanden, C. (2000) 'Gene Cheats', *New Scientist*, 24–9.

Bette, K-H. and Schimank, U. (2001) 'Coping with Doping: Sport Associations under Organizational Stress', In *Proceedings from the Work Shop Research on Doping in Sport* (22 May), pp. 51–69.

Biesta, G. (1995) 'Education/Communication. The Two Faces of Communicative Pedagogy', in A.M. Neiman (ed.) *The Philosophy of Education Society Yearbook 1995*.

Biesta, G. (1997) 'Onmogelijke opvoeding: Kanttekeningen bij de pedagogische overdrachtsmetafoor', *Comenius*, 17: 312–24.

Bouchard, C., Malina, R.M. and Pérusse, L. (1997) *Genetics of Fitness and Physical Performance*. Champaign, IL: Human Kinetics.

Breivik, G. (2000) 'Against Chance: A Causal Theory of Winning in Sport', in T. Tännsjö and C. Tamburrini (eds), *Values in Sport: Elitism, Nationalism, Gender Equality and the Scientific Manufacture of Winners*. London: E & FN Spon, pp. 141–56.

Brown, W.M. (1990) 'Practices and Prudence', *Journal of the Philosophy of Sport*, XVII: 71–84.

Buchanan, A., Brock, D.W., Daniels, N. and Wikler, D. (2000) *From Chance to Choice: Genetics and Justice*. Cambridge, Cambridge: University Press.

Campbell, A.V. (1990) 'Education or Indoctrination? The Issue of Autonomy in Health Education', in S. Doxiadis (ed.) *Ethics in Health Education*. Chichester: John Wiley & Sons, Ltd, pp. 15–27.

Cooke, E.F. (2003) 'Germ-Line Engineering, Freedom, and Future Generations', *Bioethics*, 17(1): 32–58.

Davis, D.S. (1997) 'Genetic Dilemmas and the Child's Right to an Open Future', *Hastings Center Report*, 27(2): 7–15.

Davis, D.S. (2001) *Genetic Dilemmas: Reproductive Technology, Parental Choices, and Children's Futures*. London: Routledge.

Gardner, W. (1995) 'Can Human Genetic Enhancement be Prohibited?', *The Journal of Medicine and Philosophy*, 20: 65–84.

Gugutzer, R. (2001) 'Die Fiktion des Natürlichen: Sportdoping in der reflexiven Moderne', *Soziale Welt*, 52: 219–38.

Hilvoorde, I.M. van (2001) 'Can Health in and through Sports be a Pedagogical Aim?' In J. Steenbergen, P. de Knop and A. Elling (eds) *Values and Norms in Sport: Critical Reflections on the Position and Meanings of Sport in Society*. Aken: Meyer & Meyer Sport, pp. 57–72.

Hilvoorde. I.M. van (2002) *Gatekeepers of Educational Science: Demarcation and Disciplining in Developments of Dutch Academic Pedagogy (1900–1970)*. Baarn: HBUitgevers (in Dutch).

Hilvoorde. I.M van (2003) 'Flopping, Klapping and Gene Doping: Shifting Dichotomies between "Natural" and "Artificial" in Elite Sport', paper presented at the workshop 'Extreme Bodies', University of Maastricht, 31 October–1 November.

Kant, I. (1964) *Schriften zur Anthropologie, Geschichtsphilosophie, Politik und Pädagogik*. Immanuel Kant Werke, vol. VI. W. Weischedel (ed.), Frankfurt am Main: Insel.

Loland, S. (2000) 'Justice and Game Advantage in Sporting Games', in T. Tännsjö and C. Tamburrini (eds), *Values in Sport: Elitism, Nationalism, Gender Equality and the Scientific Manufacture of Winners*. London: E & FN Spon, pp. 151–71.

Loland, S. (2002) *Fair Play in Sport: A Moral Norm System*. London: Routledge.

Magdalinski, T. and Brooks, K. (2002) 'Bride of Frankenstein: Technology and the Consumption of the Female Athlete', in A. Miah and S. Eassom (eds) *Sport Technology: History, Philosophy and Policy*. Amsterdam: Elsevier Science Ltd, pp. 195–212.

Miah, A. (2002) 'Philosophical and Ethical Questions Concerning Technology and Sport: The Case of Genetic Modification', PhD thesis, De Montfort University, Leicester.

Miah, A. and Eassom, S.B. (eds) (2002) *Sport Technology: History, Philosophy and Policy*. Amsterdam: Elsevier Science Ltd.

Montgomery, H.E. *et al.* (1998) 'Human Gene for Physical Performance', *Nature*, 393: 221–2.

Munthe, C. (2000) 'Selected Champions: Making Winners in the Age of Genetic Technology', in T. Tännsjö and C. Tamburrini (eds), *Values in Sport: Elitism, Nationalism, Gender Equality and the Scientific Manufacture of Winners*. London: E & FN Spon, pp. 217–31.

Rankinen, T., Pérusse, L., Rauramaa, R., Rivera, M., Wolfarth, B. and Bouchard, C. (2001) 'The human gene map for performance and health-related fitness phenotypes', *Medical Science of Sports and Exercise*, 33(6): 855–67.

Ruyter, D.J. de (2003) 'The Importance of Ideals in Education', *Journal of Philosophy of Education*, 37(3): 467–82.

Siegel, H. (1991) 'Indoctrination and Education', in B. Spiecker and R. Straughan (eds) *Freedom and Indoctrination in Education: International Perspectives*. London: Cassell, pp. 30–41.

Skinner, J.S. (2001) 'Do Genes Determine Champions?', *Sports Science Exchange*, 14 (4).

Soderberg, W. (1998) 'Genetic Enhancement of a Child's Memory: A Search for a Private and Public Morality', hypertext document: http://www.bu.edu/wcp/Papers/Bioe/BioeSode.htm

Spiecker, B. and Straughan, R. (eds) (1991) *Freedom and Indoctrination in Education: International Perspectives*. London: Cassell.

Steenbergen, J., Buisman, A. and van Hilvoorde, I. (2001) 'Meanings of Fair Play in Competitive Sport', in J. Steenbergen, P. de Knop and A. Elling (eds) *Values and Norms in Sport: Critical Reflections on the Position and Meanings of Sport in Society*. Aken: Meyer & Meyer Sport, pp. 137–156.

Steinacker, J.M. and Wolfarth, B. (2002) 'Molekularbiologie und Molekulargenetik: Eine zukünftige Herausforderung in der Sportmedizin', *Deutsche Zeitschrift für Sportmedizin*, 53(12): 337.

Tamburrini, C.M. (2000) *The 'Hand of God'?: Essays in the Philosophy of Sports*. Göteborg: Acta Universitatis Gothoburgensis.

Tamburrini, C.M. (2002) 'After Doping, What? The Morality of the Genetic Engineering of Athletes', in A. Miah and S. Eassom (eds) *Sport Technology: History, Philosophy and Policy*. Amsterdam: Elsevier Science Ltd.

Tofler, I.R., Katz Stryer, B., Micheli, L.J. and Herman, L.R. (1996) 'Physical and Emotional Problems of Elite Female Gymnasts', *The New England Journal of Medicine*, 335(4): 281–3.

Tymowski, G. (1999) 'An Ethical Consideration of the Participation of Children in High-Performance Sport', Proceedings of the 7th Annual International Olympic Academic Post Graduate Seminar, Athens, Greece.

Wadler, G.I. (1999) 'Doping in Sport: From Strychnine to Genetic Enhancement, It's a Moving Target', paper presented at the Duke Conference on Doping in Sport, Durham, North Carolina, 7/8 May.

Wijsbek, H. (2000) 'The Pursuit of Beauty: The Enforcement of Aesthetics or a Freely Adopted Lifestyle?', *Journal of Medical Ethics*, 26: 454–8.

Wolfarth, B. (2002) 'Genetische Polymorphismen bei hochtrainierten Ausdauerathleten: die Genathlete-Studie', *Deutsche Zeitschrift für Sportmedizin*, 53(12): 338–44.

Part III
Genetic testing of athletes

9 Ethical aspects of controlling genetic doping

Christian Munthe

INTRODUCTION

The continued successful development of the science and technology of genetics, combined with the evaluative and motivational forces at work in elite sports, makes it increasingly likely that, in the not too distant future, gene technology will be used for the purpose of enhancing the various performance capacities of elite athletes.[1] In response to this prospect, the international elite sports movement has recently decided on a strong commitment to fight such uses of gene technology – so-called gene doping. In a statement from a conference on genetic enhancement of athletic performance arranged by the World Anti-doping Agency (WADA) in 2002, it was said that: 'WADA is committed to confronting the possible misuse of gene transfer technology in sport. The same kinds of people who cheat in sport today will probably try to find ways to misuse genetics tomorrow'[2] and that, therefore,

> There are evident risks that genetic transfer technologies might be used in a manner that would be contrary to the spirit of sport or potentially dangerous to the health of athletes. Akin to doping in the present generation, genetic transfer technology that is non-therapeutic and merely performance-enhancing should be prohibited.[3]

In consequence, the updated 2003 version of the Anti-Doping Code of the Olympic Movement now includes among its listed 'prohibited methods' the item 'gene doping'. This, in turn, is defined as the 'non-therapeutic use of genes, genetic elements and/or cells that have the capacity to enhance athletic performance.'[4] Obviously, if this commitment to the fight against gene doping is to have any force, it must also include the aim of developing control programmes for the detection of gene doping in athletes. This issue was also addressed at the above-mentioned WADA conference and it was stated that:

> The scientific community has recognized the need for the continued development and refinement of methods that will permit the detection of the

misuse of genetic transfer technologies in sport. The conference noted there are a number of approaches that currently exist, or are in development, that will permit such detection.[5]

And, furthermore, that: 'The present focus of WADA's research grants toward the study of the detection methods for the misuse of oxygen carrying agents and growth factors should be extended to include the detection of genetic transfer technologies and their effects.'[6] As a consequence of this, in recent communications, WADA has announced the availability of funds for the research on and development of detection methods that may be used in control programmes for gene doping.[7]

In this chapter, I will outline and, to some extent, address the ethical implications of this development. The reason for highlighting this aspect is that the methods for detecting gene doping will necessarily have to include procedures of genetic testing, i.e., the detection of genetic sequences within athletes. Without doubt, it is such procedures that are alluded to when, in the quotation above, WADA talked about 'a number of approaches that currently exist, or are in development, that will permit such detection [of gene doping]'. However, since the practice of genetic testing within medicine and health care has come to actualize a number of hard ethical issues, this means that the international sports movement are seriously contemplating the use of ethically controversial medical procedures on perfectly healthy people. Thus, it is a matter of urgency to consider to what extent this ethical controversy can be predicted to extend also to such uses, and what implications this will have for the question of what ethical requirements must be met by a control programme for gene doping, in order for it to be a defensible practice. Procedures and programmes for doping control have until now been treated mainly as an internal affair of the sports community (controversies having to do mainly with the reliability of tests and the handling of conflicts between anti-doping regulation and the legislation of individual countries). In contrast, the newly adopted stance on gene doping necessitates the adoption of a broader perspective, where general considerations of medical ethics (and regulations based on that) are taken heavily into account when designing the envisioned handling of gene doping. Otherwise, not only will the activity of gene doping control be morally unjustified, it will be unjustified for the very same reason used when advocating that gene doping should be banned – namely, that it constitutes a serious misuse of medical technology.

I will start in the next section by outlining the various forms of genetic interventions that might be considered to fall under the new ban, to what extent it is realistic to believe these forms are detectable and what is required of a control programme to secure such detection to a sufficient degree. The conclusion is that the kind of gene doping that may be reasonable to target both from the perspective of general anti-doping ideology and that of practicality is the so-called somatic genetic modification of athletes. Moreover, it is argued that the envisioned possibilities of detetcting this form of gene doping presented by WADA and the Olympic Movement are overly optimistic and simplified. Reliable control programmes will have to include quite extensive procedures of repeated sample taking and genetic mapping of athletes.

In the third section, I will proceed by giving a brief overview of the ethical issues of genetic testing arising in the context of health care. In connection to that, I will also present some standard views (and arguments supporting these) present within medical ethics as to what requirements must be met by genetic testing programmes in the health care setting in order for these to be morally acceptable. Some important similarities and differences between the case of genetic testing for disease (or predisposition for disease) and the case of such testing being undertaken with the purpose of detecting gene doping in the elite sports context will be noted.

Finally, I will sum up my conclusions regarding the extent to which the ethical issues of genetic testing in the health care setting are relevant for gene doping control programmes and what this implies regarding moral requirements that have to be met. It is argued that while some of the problems of genetic testing for disease seem to be much less troublesome when considering the detection of gene doping, others are instead becoming significantly more serious. I conclude that considerations from medical ethics seem to imply that control programmes for gene doping will have to be much more complicated and expensive than the more traditional anti-doping procedures. Moreover, ethical considerations speak strongly in favour of the claim that some degree of reliability in such control programmes will have to be sacrificed if they are to be ethically defensible.

GENETIC INTERVENTIONS: PROSPECTS OF DETECTION

In order to correctly assess the prospects of detecting gene doping, it is necessary to begin by considering what kind of genetic interventions may be taken to be covered by the newly adopted ban. Unfortunately, however, already at this basic level, the understanding within the international elite sports community of what genetic interventions may amount to and, in fact, how genes function seems to be seriously lacking. For if we reconsider the Olympic Movement's definition of gene doping in the quotation above – the 'non-therapeutic use of genes, genetic elements and/or cells that have the capacity to enhance athletic performance' – and take it literally, it would seem to ban all athletic activity. This is due to the elementary fact that genes, genetic elements and cells are natural entities present in all living organisms and governing their functions whatever these are – hence also the performance of any athlete. However, to be a bit more charitable, what the definition is supposed to say is obviously that it is the use of *artificially modified* genes, genetic elements or cells that are prohibited. In effect, a reliable control programme for gene doping must be able to detect not only genes etc., but also the presence of artificially modified elements of this kind. The importance of including the requirement of artificiality here is that the ban is surely not intended to stop athletes from competing because they happen to have been subject to natural mutations (i.e. changes in their genetic make-up caused by something else than human intervention, such as radiation, toxic exposure or viral infection). In conclusion, therefore, any method for detecting gene doping must be able to distinguish between atheletes who have an enhanced capacity for performance due to (1) their natural genetic make-up; (2) a genetic make-up changed by natural causes; and (3) a genetic make-up modified through human intervention.[8]

As a direct consequence of this, the implied optimism in the quotation above talking about existing metothods that permit the detection of gene doping is hardly warranted. These methods all amount to the same thing, namely producing information about the genetic make-up of an individual through some sort of genetic testing procedure. In the case when one knows that a genetic modification of such an individual has been attempted (as in the case of research on gene therapy), such methods may be used for investigating whether or not the modification attempt has been successful. One simply examines whether or not the desired end result is present within the genetic make-up. However, this method lacks any capacity to distinguish between different reasons for the presence of any given genetic variant, should this be unknown. In elite sports, we may plausibly expect most top athletes to be equipped with a genetic make-up that, in comparison to the average person, may be labelled as performance-enhancing (this is what explains their initial talent for sports). Therefore, to discover such genetic variants will be quite far from discovering any gene doping. In order to do that, the methods must be able not only to discover genetic variants with performance-enhancing functions, they must also be able to separate the above mentioned cases (1) and (2) from (3) – where only (3) would indicate a case of gene doping.

Bearing these complications in mind, let us now take a look at the chief possibilities of genetic intervention that may hope to count as artificial modification of the kind that is (or, rather, should be) covered by the gene doping ban.[9]

The first family of interventions is the use of genetic testing for selection purposes. Testing procedures of this kind are already a reality and are applied in health care for a variety of purposes and in different stages of human development, from gametes to grown-ups. The testing itself reveals genetic information about individuals – in this case, information of relevance for athletic performance capacities – and this information can, in turn, be used as a basis for selective decisions regarding single individuals or within groups, such as who is to be given the opportunity to develop his or her capacity for athletic achievement. The most obvious example of this would be the selection among promising and seemingly talented junior athletes as to who among these would be further supported by sports organizations, sponsors, etc. However, the selection may also take place before birth, pregnancy or even conception – thereby constituting a preselection of foetuses, embryos or gametes with elevated genetic potentials to give rise to an individual with enhanced capacities for athletic performance.[10]

It seems quite clear that none of these interventions could ever be detected. A genetic test may, of course, reveal that an individual is a carrier of a genetic trait that enhances athletic performance capacities. However, this says absolutely nothing about whether or not he or she has been the subject of a genetically informed selection or preselection procedure. At the same time, however, this may not be such a big worry, since it seems quite plausible to argue that such interventions should not be counted as gene doping anyway (although that is not made clear by the newly adopted ban). For, in spite of the fact that these kind of interventions may be very powerful indeed in producing individuals with elevated athletic performance capacities, they do not involve any modification of the initial genetic make-up of any of these individuals. They merely amount to choosing among them on the basis of knowledge about this make-up.

The second family of interventions consists of using methods of so-called germ-line gene therapy to produce inheritable changes of the genome built into the initial genetic make-up of individuals. Although applied to various types of animals and plants, such modifications have not yet been attempted on human beings[11] and are also, at the present stage, viewed as ethically very controversial. However, with time, it is not unreasonable to expect such methods will be developed and refined in the context of medical research on genetic disease. And, once they are, there seems to be no further technical or scientific barrier impeding their application for the purpose of producing individuals with increased genetic capacities for athletic performance.

Also in this case, the prospects of detecting genetic interventions seem to be rather slim. Again, it is, of course, quite possible to use genetic testing to detect the presence within an individual of genetic variants that increase athletic performance capacities. But, as before, this will in itself not reveal anything about the reason for the presence of such genetic variants. Since the result of a germ-line genetic modification will be built into the individual's initial genetic make-up, a genetic test will be unable to tell us whether an individual has this genetic make-up due to natural causes or some kind of germ-line genetic intervention. To complicate things even further, since this kind of genetic modification is inheritable, the individual that carries a genetic variant that has been introduced through such modification may not have been subject to such a procedure him or herself – not even at the gamete stage. He or she may simply have inherited it from his or her parents (who, in turn, have been genetically modified or inherited the genetic variant from their parents who have been modified, etc.).[12] Again, however, although this is a bit more controversial than in the case of genetically informed selection, there appears to be quite strong reasons to claim that these kinds of interventions should not be counted as gene doping at all. To be valid, an artificial procedure must have been applied and this procedure has introduced a genetic variant that would otherwise not have been present. In this sense, we are dealing with artificially modified genes, genetic elements, etc. However, it is much harder to claim that this modification has been made on any specific individual and that this individual, therefore, has had his or her athletic performance capacities enhanced. Rather, what has been achieved is the construction of one specific individual with one specific genetic make-up rather than another individual who would have had another genetic make-up.[13] Or, at least, what has been achieved is the construction of an individual including his or her initial genetic make-up. In any case, it would seem impossible to speak about any modification of this individual's initial genetic make-up having taken place.

This brings us to the third and last family of interventions, so-called somatic genetic modification. In this case we are dealing with modifications that clearly change an individual's intial genetic make-up and, moreover, modifications that affect only specific parts of the human body (although these may be parts that, in turn, have a widespread influence on this individual's physical capabilities – such as bone marrow cells governing the production of components of the blood). In this case, the present stage of development can be called very experimental but much less of science fiction than in the case of germ-line genetic modification procedures. As in the case with germ-line gene therapy, we may safely expect that when we have reliable procedures for somatic genetic gene therapy, some people will be very prepared indeed to use these for somatic gene doping purposes. Somatic genetic modification may be achieved either through direct modification of the genome of the cells of an individual or through transplantation of 'foreign' cells that may or may not have been subject to genetic modification.[14] Moreover, and more important in the present context, the modifications may be introduced either in their 'natural' place in the body (modified muscle cells within the muscles, modified blood cells in the blood, etc.) or as 'depots' of modified or 'foreign' cells producing natural bodily substances that enhance athletic performance capacities. These depots can then, in turn, be 'hidden' in suitable places within the body – such as deep inside any of the great muscles of the buttocks (musculus gluteus maximus).[15]

Although the possibility of this last strategy of hidden depots creates serious complications, in contrast to the aforementioned types of genetic intervention, detection of somatic genetic modifications seems to be a definite feasibility from a purely technical point of view. Again, of course, mere detection of a genetic variant with the potential of enhancing athletic performance capacities will not do. However, in the case of somatic modifications there is something to compare with, namely those parts of the individual's body that have not been genetically modified. The most straightforward strategy here would seem to be to take cell samples from those body parts most likely to be tampered with and compare the genetic make-up of these with other parts of the body. In order to know the original genetic make-up of the individual, this procedure presupposes that the complete genome has been scanned quite early on (preferably in childhood or early adolescence when the use of somatic gene doping is still quite unlikely). If this has been done and if a genetic aberration is found that is also in favour of the individual's chances of athletic achievement, it may be concluded that a case of gene doping has been detected.[16] However, the risk of missing those cells that have undergone modification would seem to be quite high and if we add the possibility of the hidden depot strategy, it would seem that even minor chances of detection would have to involve very extensive sample taking indeed. Not only would tissue samples have to be taken from a whole collection of different body parts, the hidden depot strategy would force very many samples to be taken from each such part in order to secure a reasonable chance of detecting hidden depots of genetically modified cells. Moreover, since a modification could occur at any time, reliable detection chances would seem to presuppose that this procedure be repeated quite often.

Now, sometime in the future it may become possible to increase the reliability of detection while actually reducing the amount of sample-taking. This could be achieved when genetic knowledge has developed so far as to permit predictions for any genetic variant (or, rather, genetic make-up) what bodily substances it will and will not produce. On this basis, it would in theory be possible to say whether or not the presence of a particular bodily substance is consistent with the genetic make-up of a person. Should this possibility become feasible, there would no longer be a need for actual sampling of the genetically modified cells – it would suffice to measure the presence of the substances produced by these cells and discover if this measure is inconsistent with the individual's initial genetic make-up.[17] However, apart from the sample-taking that would still have to be performed in order to detect the bodily substances to be compared to the individual's genome, this strategy would presuppose very detailed analysis of the individual's complete genetic make-up that may be expected to reveal a lot of things about him or her that has nothing to do with doping or athletic performance capacity. Although this information would be produced also by the initial genome scan presupposed in the more basic method involving much more sample-taking described above, in that case the information would to a large extent merely be latent and possible to decipher only when genetic research had made the advances presupposed in this latter sketch of a detection method. It should be observed, however, that also a complete genome scan done on the basis of present genetic knowledge would produce quite large quantities of information of no relevance to sport but of clear relevance to the individual in question, such as information on genetic predispositions for various diseases and corresponding hereditary risks to the offspring of the athlete.

THE ETHICS OF GENETIC TESTING: A CRASH COURSE

Let me now move on to give a brief overview of the main ethical issues arising in the area of genetic testing in the health care setting.[18] In passing, I will also make some comments on the applicability of these issues to the case of genetic testing for the purpose of detecting gene doping.

Risks and problems involved in sample-taking

First, we have issues regarding the safety of and possible problems with the taking of bodily samples necessary for any genetic analysis. In the health care context, this issue arises mostly in the areas of prenatal and pre-implantation genetic diagnosis, where the sample-taking involves advanced invasive procedures penetrating the uterus of a pregnant woman or the inner cell mass of an early embryo and thereby presenting peculiar risks of, for example, miscarriage. Otherwise, however, the sample-taking needed for genetic testing (i.e., that performed on people) is no more risky or burdensome than the taking of a regular blood sample. In some cases, it may actually cause even less inconvenience, since our DNA may be analysed many times from cells, the collection of which do not require penetration of the skin. For this reason, risks in and possible problems with sample-taking have not been much of an issue in the ethical discussion of genetic testing on people.

However, in light of what has been outlined in the preceding section, it would seem that genetic testing for the purpose of detecting gene doping is a radically different case. Due to the apparent need for quite extensive and repeated sample-taking, health risks due to the repeated application of biopsy procedures to various parts of the body have to be taken quite seriously. The same goes, of course, for the direct and rather obvious inconvenience of the athlete who has to be subjected to such procedures. Any programme for controlling gene doping would therefore have to consider the risks and problems created by the sample-taking alone as an ethically highly relevant factor that needs to balanced against the reasons for enforcing and upholding the ban on gene doping.

Reliability of results

This brings us immediately to the next issue, since a key element of any successful control programme for gene doping is the reliability of applied detection methods. The issue of reliability is also a key issue in the ethics of genetic testing in the health care context, since reduced reliability always brings risks of missing either the presence of disease or risk thereof (so-called false negatives) or its non-presence (so-called false positives). While it may be seen as a serious flaw in itself that patients are given false information, what is much worse, this in turn brings serious risks of important decisions being based on such faulty information – in the worst case with fatal results.

In the context of detecting gene doping, such drastic scenarios do not seem very relevant. However, the reliability of applied detection methods is still an issue from an ethical point of view in at least three ways. Moreover, these ways seem to pull in slightly different directions as to what they imply regarding desirable features of a gene doping control programme.

First, since the aim of the programme is to provide information that will be used in decisions about the application of various anti-doping sanctions, basic considerations of judicial security require that applied testing procedures have a very high reliability in the sense of not missing the non-presence of artificially modified genes (i.e., of avoiding false positives). Second, since the aim of the control programme is to fight the use of gene doping as efficiently as possible, applied testing procedures need to have a very high reliability in the sense of avoiding false negatives, that is, of not missing the presence of artificially modified genes that enhance athletic performance capacities. However, since this last requirement would seem to imply the need to include testing also when the result of the test does not unequivocally indicate the presence of such genes (but only makes it a bit likely), there is a conflict between this second requirement regarding the efficiency in the fight against gene doping and the first requirement regarding the judicial security of athletes.[19] Third, due to the possible strategies of gene doping mentioned above, high reliability in the sense of avoiding false negatives would seem to require quite extensive procedures of sample-taking. However, this, as we have already seen, may lead to conflicts with considerations regarding the medical safety and other problems for the athletes.

In all, this situation highlights the fact that the decision regarding what tests to actually include in a control programme for gene doping has to be made on the basis of a delicate balance of ethically highly relevant considerations regarding legitimate claims on behalf of athletes and the value of a successful prevention of gene doping. This balance may seem comparable to the balance between the value of avoiding false negatives and that of avoiding false positives in the health care context. However, while in health care the concern for avoiding false positives only has to do with the importance of avoiding negative effects on patients effected by the false belief that they are afflicted by disease (such as fear, anxiety and the application of unnecessary medical procedures), in the sports context we also have to add the legitimate interest of athletes not to be subjected to anti-doping sanctions in the absence of adequate proofs of guilt. Moreover, while in the health care case the importance of avoiding false negatives has to do with the rather serious possibility of people contracting diseases or missing possible treatment options, in the sports context what is risked is merely that a number of athletes may get away with cheating.

Risks of misunderstanding

A central element in ethical discussions of genetic testing is the concern for the patient's ability to understand the information produced by such a test. This, in turn, has to do with three different factors. First, when used in the health care context, the general value of genetic testing is that it may provide information about the presence or non-presence of some particular disease (or risk thereof) that is more precise and accurate than the information that may be obtained by other means. This is of value since such information may be used by the patient to improve his or her decision-making regarding the application of medical procedures or various health-related 'life-style choices'. Second, the information regarding the nature of a detected disease and the pros and cons of available medical procedures that may be used for counteracting this disease may be highly complex and ambiguous and, therefore, hard to comprehend even for a medical specialist. Third, in most cases, the information provided by a genetic test will be ambiguous, since it will only say something about the likelihood of contracting this or that disease. Moreover, when the heredity of the trait tested for is complex (or, as it is sometimes called, polygenetic), this information regarding likelihood will be very complicated and difficult to interpret. In all, then, although a genetic test may in theory provide information that helps the patient to make better-informed decisions, in practice, the complexity of the information may in fact make more confusion than clarification. In effect, the patient's ability to predict the consequences of different choices may actually be impaired rather than strengthened by a genetic test. These problems are further accentuated by the fact that these patients are often afflicted by emotional stress, anxiety, guilt feelings towards relatives and similar states that further impair their capacity both to adequately comprehend the information provided by a test and to relate this information to a clear conception of what they want to achieve in the choices that are actualized by this information.

Now, in the gene doping context, the situation may seem to be radically different. Here, the purpose and value of genetic tests are not to help guide the decision making of athletes, but to detect the illegitimate use of genetic modification. In the course of this, it may be discovered that an athlete carries a genetic trait that enhances athletic performance capacities (be it present due to natural causes or due to some form of gene doping). This, however, does not seem to actualize any important decisions on the part of the athlete on a par with, for example, the choice between medical procedures aimed at preventing a grave disease. At worst, a misunderstanding of the test result may make the athlete overconfident regarding his or her inborn talent for sports. Of course, the test may instead reveal that the athlete in question lacks such traits and this may actualize the question of whether or not he or she should continue a career in elite sports. In this case, a misunderstanding may cause the athlete to needlessly disrupt his or her career due to exaggerated interpretations of the implications of the test result, or, conversely, to hopelessly continue the struggle to reach the top due to lack of understanding of the significance of genetic traits for athletic performance. Again, however, none of these worst-case scenarios seem even remotely comparable to the kind of choices and possible negative effects of misunderstandings of test results that are actualized in the health care context. For this reason, then, the risk that the athlete does not fully comprehend the information provided by a genetic test undertaken in the context of a programme for controlling gene doping may appear to provide no grounds for ethically relevant concern. This, however, is a premature conclusion that rests on a grave simplification of the nature of genetic information.

Additional information

While the information sought by a gene doping control programme is not in itself relevant for any important decisions on behalf of the athlete, the information provided by a genetic test made in order to detect gene doping may always produce additional information that is relevant for this. This is true also of genetic testing in the health care context. However, while in that context it merely adds to the ethical concerns that are already present regarding possible misunderstandings, in the sports context it radically changes the situation regarding such concerns.

Already today, it is well known that some genetic traits that may enhance athletic performance capacities also bring peculiar health risks. Testing for such traits will therefore produce information of direct relevance to health. Moreover, even if this is not the case, genetic traits that may enhance athletic performance capacities are almost always peculiar variants (or mutations) of genes that in other variants may cause impairment or disease. This means that if an athlete is aware of the presence of hereditary pathological traits in his or her family, and the gene doping test produces information regarding the non-presence of such a trait, the above-mentioned peculiar guilt feelings towards those relatives that carry the trait may be actualized.

These aspects may seem serious enough. However, if we consider what was said in the preceding section regarding the need for complete genome scans and extensive sample-taking in order to secure the reliability of applied detection methods, the seriousness of the problems of this kind actualized by a control programme for gene doping seems to expand exponentially. For if such measures are applied, it is unavoidable that they will produce vast amounts of genetic information about athletes of direct relevance to their health. This includes information about causes of pathologies from which the athlete suffers, elevated vulnerability in the face of various environmental exposures (such as toxic substances, drugs, and particular types of food) and, most important, elevated risks of contracting various diseases. Already today, quite a lot is known about genetic factors connected to such phenomena. However, as research in genetics and medicine proceeds further, we may safely expect that in the future this body of knowledge will expand considerably.

The consequence of all this seems to be that the likelihood of misunderstandings of genetic information produced by a control programme for gene doping that may have serious consequences increases drastically. Such a programme will inevitably make athletes vulnerable to more or less the same risks of misunderstanding as in the health care context. Moreover, in the sports context, this risk actually seems to be greater, since the athlete subjected to a gene doping test is not prepared to receive health-related information in the same way as a patient in the health care setting who undergoes a genetic test because of initial health-related worries. Besides being serious as such, these facts also add to the above mentioned tension between the concern of efficiency of control programmes for gene doping and the concern of not harming athletes.

Third party interests

One peculiar family of issues in ethical debates about genetic testing is related to the fact that the information produced by such tests is of considerable interest not only to the person being tested, but also to various third parties. The most obvious of these are the relatives of the tested person. If a test reveals the presence of a health-related genetic trait in an individual, this immediately implies that the relatives of this individual have elevated risks of carrying the same trait. The question then arises whether or not these relatives can be said to have a legitimate claim to the information in question and, if so, how one should handle the not very uncommon phenomenon of people who do not wish their relatives to be informed about the result after having been subjected to a genetic test. On the one hand, informing the relatives in such cases may be seen as a serious invasion of the privacy of the patient through the compromising of the integrity of patient records. On the other, the very fact that the patient is given the information from the genetic test means that he or she receives genetic information about his or her relatives without their prior consent. Moreover, if the relatives are informed, it may turn out that they do not want this information and consider this act an invasion of their privacy. However, whether or not they actually will react in that way is impossible to know beforehand. In practice, many clinics where genetic testing is performed try to handle this problem by handing it over to the patient. However, this increases the risk of the patient not informing relatives who for good reasons would have preferred to be informed. Moreover, if the patient does choose to inform relatives, the risk of serious misunderstandings increases, since the patient is not an expert on the subject. Finally, this strategy in no way makes the aforementioned ethical problems disappear – it merely shifts the burden of responsibility from health care to the patient – and it may plausibly be argued that health care is still responsible for the possible unethical results of this shift.

Besides relatives, there are also a number of other parties who have an interest in the information produced by genetic tests. The most obvious of these are insurance companies providing life and health-insurance policies. First, if these companies are allowed to demand genetic tests, they can adapt the insurance premiums to reflect the actual risks of the individual insurance-holders in a more adequate way. This obviously brings the risk that those who are most in need of insurance cannot have it, since it will be too expensive or since the companies will refuse them insurance altogether. Second, if insurance-holders are allowed to have genetic tests without revealing the results of these, they may use this information for a peculiar form of insurance scams. Knowing that they have a high risk of contracting some disease in the future they may buy a life or health-insurance policy with a very high return without having to pay the high premium that would reflect their actual risk. This, in turn, forces insurance companies to raise premiums for all insurance-holders in order to avoid bankrupcy. If some companies are allowed to demand such information and some are not, the result will then be that the latter companies will eventually lose those customers who know themselves to be at low risk for contracting genetic diseases to the former companies, which in turn will leave the latter companies in an impossible situation, where also those who have high risks of contracting genetic diseases will lose their insurance coverage. If, instead, these companies are allowed to demand such information, the result will be the same: those who run high risks will be left without insurance coverage due to high premiums or refusal of insurance altogether. This has been put forward as a reason for an obligation of those who have genetic tests that indicate elevated risks of disease to reveal this information to insurance companies. However, again, this will mean that many of these people will be left without insurance altogether. True, they may avoid this risk by abstaining from having genetic tests. However, since such tests may be very beneficial to them in terms of health, this may be seen as too high a price to require them to pay.

At the moment the situation regarding regulations that affect this problem is varying across the world and seems also to be very dynamic. This regards not least the possibility of individuals who are unable to obtain private insurance to cover their losses by seeking help from systems of publicly financed health insurance. There is a rapid development in the West where such systems are being gradually deconstructed to the benefit of privately financed insurance and this, of course, sharpens the seriousness of the issues mentioned above.[20] Moreover, the case of insurance companies will most likely soon be complemented by the interest of employers to avoid an unhealthy workforce – especially so if employers (as is often the case) are responsible for paying the insurance premiums of employees in a predominantly private system of health insurance.

From the point of view of programmes for controlling gene doping, this complex of problems is actualized mainly due to the phenomenon of additional information. Since the gene doping tests will unavoidably produce health-related information about athletes, the latter will be exposed to the various risks arising out of the interest in this information from various third parties. Moreover, sports officials will therefore have to consider the peculiar issue of whether or not the results of tests should be revealed to such third parties when requested. In the case of tests done within health care, the normal procedure is that the tested individual is the owner of the information produced by the test. Therefore, if he or she agrees to the right of, for example, an insurance company to inspect his or her medical records, health care has no right to refuse. But records of doping tests are usually surrounded by much more secrecy and it is therefore far from clear how these should be handled in similar situations.

Informed consent

One important conclusion reached within health care on the basis of all the aspects mentioned above is that an ethically acceptable practice of genetic testing presupposes that tested individuals have given their informed consent. Basically, this involves four separate things. First, the individual is ascribed an absolute right to refuse testing. Second, he or she is ascribed a similar right to abandon an initiated testing procedure at any stage. For example, the individual may take the test, but refuse to be informed about the results or about some particular part of these results. Third, this right can be exercised without any adverse consequences besides the possible loss of benefits that would have resulted from the testing itself. That is, refusal of testing or abandonment of an initiated testing procedure must in no way affect the access to other benefits, such as health care and social support. Fourth, the individual has a right to be provided with accurate, comprehensible and sufficiently substantial information about their rights and the various risks and possible benefits of testing in order for the individual to be able to make a rational decision as to whether or not to undergo it. The underlying rationale for the informed consent model is that it must be up to the affected individual to assess and evaluate whether or not the various risks of a particular genetic testing procedure are worth taking in light of its possible benefits. After all, it is this individual and no one else who will have to live with the result of accepting or refusing an offer to undergo a test.

In light of what has been said above about the extent to which atheletes undergoing genetic testing in a doping control setting will be exposed to the prospects and dangers facing people who undergo genetic testing in a health care context, the rationale of the informed consent model seems to be at least as applicable to the former group as it is to the latter. However, at the same time, the setting of doping control within an elite sports context makes the full application of informed consent impossible. For, in this setting, if someone refuses to participate in the programme, the rule that access to other benefits must not be affected by such a decision will not be in effect. On the contrary, athletes who refuse to take the required tests in a doping control programme will normally be punished by temporal or permanent expulsion from competition.

It may be argued that this breach of the basic requirements of informed consent is not that serious. After all, athletes are not in the situation of a patient who depends on health care for upholding a minimally decent quality of life. To be true, an elite athlete often makes a living from his or her athletic achievements, however, in most cases, could surely just as well make a living from something else instead. Of course, choosing another profession may mean some loss of benefits, however, the seriousness of this loss comes no way near that of the loss affecting a patient in health care who is deprived of access to further care. Nevertheless, even though it may in the just indicated way be possible to make a case for the acceptability of such a practice, it is no doubt that a control programme for gene doping will mean that people are pressured into undergoing medical procedures associated with a rather large number of risk scenarios.

However, even if this is accepted, there remain the other requirements of informed consent. First, there is no reason why, in the anti-doping context, atheletes should be deprived of the right to decide for themselves, on the basis of accurate and relevant information, whether or not to participate in a doping control programme. Of course, should they come to the decision not to participate, this will mean giving up their athletic career, but then at least they have made this decision themselves on the basis of information that provides a picture of risks and possible benefits that is accurate and relevant. Furthermore, regarding genetic testing in a doping control context in particular, there remain very good reasons indeed for giving tested athletes the opportunity of deciding for themselves what in the results of the tests they are to be informed about (not counting, of course, the detection or non-detection of gene doping). Again, this presupposes access to accurate and relevant information in light of which people may make rational decisions about such matters.

Genetic counselling

What has just been said implies that a minimal requirement that must be met by any gene doping control programme in order for it to be ethically defensible is that it provides a set-up for informing athletes about the purpose and set-up of the programme, as well as the various risks and possible benefits associated with participation or non-participation. This, however, involves a whole body of further ethical issues. For it is a long-standing lesson from the field of genetic testing in health care that providing such information in a way that actually promotes rational decision-making is not an easy task. The collected experience on this has provided the foundation for what is nowadays usually referred to as genetic counselling, i.e., the peculiar art of informing people about genetic matters and procedures, and taking care of them in an appropriate way in connection to this, in order to actually promote their chances of making rational decisions about things related to such information.

I will not go into the various difficulties involved in genetic counselling, but merely point to the fact demonstrated above that the possible implications of taking or not taking a genetic test may be highly complex and involve a number of other hard choices. Issues about risky medical treatments, family relations or whether or not to have children, as well as such things as the ability to get a job or being able to purchase health insurance, are all relevant when facing the choice of whether or not to take a genetic test. As we have seen above, despite the initial appearance that gene doping tests would not involve such matters, in fact, they would have to if they are going to be minimally efficient.

The lesson learned within genetic counselling is primarily that this activity requires quite a lot of time and resources. A tentative conclusion would therefore seem to be that if gene doping control programmes are to be ethically justified, they will at least have to be much more time-consuming and expensive than envisaged in the minds of those sports officials supporting the ban on gene doping.

WHAT IS GOOD ENOUGH TO OFFER?

This takes us to the final of those ethical issues arising in the field of genetic testing in health care on which I will comment. For, on the basis of all those other issues that have been described above, it is always an open question whether a certain genetic test should be offered or not. Furthermore, the decision to offer such a test is open to moral criticism if the test can be shown not to be 'good enough'. As a general possibility regarding all medical procedures, assessing whether or not a genetic test is good enough, of course, includes balancing its risks and possible benefits. However, as we have seen above, the possible risks associated with genetic tests go far beyond the possibility of direct and simple physical injury. For this reason, in many cases, health care may decide not to offer genetic tests that are from a narrow medical perspective not very dangerous. This is due to the large number of secondary risks associated with the phenomena of misunderstanding and additional information, as well as the problems involved of providing appropriate genetic counselling.

These decisions are taken despite the fact that the tests may also provide some medical benefits. However, in the case of gene doping control programmes, the benefits of the tests are not even medical. They are about upholding and enforcing a rule within the peculiar field of elite sports. On this basis, it does not seem unreasonable to conclude that normal medical ethical reasoning would not approve of the use of several genetic tests in this area, although these may be approved in a health care setting. Or, at least, such reasoning would require much more limitations and safeguards than would be required in a health care context.

CONCLUSION

It may, of course, be questioned why the international elite sports community should worry about standards and values adopted and developed in the health care context. After all, elite sports is a world of its own and in many ways it may seem to celebrate values and virtues quite opposed to that of medicine and care. However, when the sports community starts to incorporate and advocate the use of medical procedures, it may be argued that considerations of medical ethics become paramount. To this may be added that one powerful reason put forward in official anti-doping statements, including those concerning gene doping, refer to doping procedures as a misuse of health care resources. If the sports community embarks on control programmes for gene doping without taking into serious consideration those aspects related in this chapter, it may quite reasonably be claimed that such programmes would be at least as much of a misuse of health care resources as would gene doping itself.

Summarizing what has been concluded above, the most important lesson seems to be that considerations of medical ethics make a strong case for the claim that a maximally efficient control programme for gene doping is impossible to justify from an ethical point of view. First, there seem to be powerful reasons supporting the suggestion that at least some of the reliability of such a programme would have to be sacrificed. Second, equally powerful arguments support the requirement that an ethically defensible programme of this sort would need to include procedures for genetic counselling and informed consent that will require quite a lot of time, manpower and, therefore, money. Some of the aspects necessitating such steps may be avoided, but then the reliability of the programme would be significantly affected for the worse. On top of that, sports officials will have to consider appropriate policies regarding the handling of genetic information resulting from such a programme, for example, in relation to the interest of insurance companies.

If the international sports community continues to follow the route relating to gene doping on which it has embarked, it is of considerable importance that the discussion of the ethical implications is given a high priority. If not, not only will this run contary to values that are condoned by the rest of society, as well as this community itself, but the programmes designed to protect the dignity of the institution of elite sports will run evident risks of causing serious harm to many athletes as well as their relatives.

ACKNOWLEDGEMENTS

The work on this chapter has been undertaken within the research project 'Genetic Counselling and Presymptomatic Genetic Testing: Goals and Ethics for Clinical Practice, Caring and Education'. I am grateful to the Swedish Ethics in Health Care Programme for the generous funding of this project. The first draft of the chapter was presented at the conference 'Gene Technology in Elite Sports', May 22–23 2003, Stockholm. I am grateful to the organizers of this conference for inviting me and, in particular, to the participants for comments and questions that have made several substantial improvements to the chapter.

NOTES

1 In a recent overview by leading experts in the field (Pérusse *et al.*, 2003), it is reported that the number of genes identified to have some type of relevance to physical performance has increased from 29 in 2000 to 106 in 2002 – and this in spite of the fact that there are still large portions of the human genome left unaccounted for. Various ways in which such knowledge may be used for the enhancement of athletic performance capacities and reasons for why these will quite likely be used when technically feasible are described in Munthe (2000, 2002).

2 WADA statement available at: http://www.wada-ama.org/en/t3.asp?p=29627&x =1&a=58573 (16 June 2003).

3 Ibid.

4 'Olympic Movement Anti-doping Code, Appendix A: Prohibited Classes of Substances and Prohibited Methods 2003', available at http://multimedia.olympic.org/pdf/en_ report_542.pdf (accessed June 16, 2003).

5 See note 2.

6 Ibid.

7 Available at: http://www.wada-ama.org/en/t3.asp?p=31748, and http://www.wada-ama.org/en/t3.asp?p=31750 (accessed 16 June 2003).

8 A further problem, of course, is to draw the line between therapeutic and non-therapeutic modifications. However, this problem is less of a technical nature, but rather has to do with the problem of distinguishing clearly between normality and pathology on the conceptual level.

9 I am here building heavily on Munthe (2000), and, to some extent, also Munthe (2002).

10 See Munthe (1999a), for more about such possibilities, as well as the ethical issues arising due to these.

11 Actually, one such attempt has been reported. However, this attempt did not involve changes of that part of the DNA residing within the nucleus of our cells, but rather the so-called mitochondrial DNA, which resides in the plasma of the cell, outside of the nucleus, and governs some basic functions of the energy supply and transport of the cell (see Barritt *et al.*, 2001). Changes to this form of DNA will not be inheritable in the simple way as other germ-line genetic changes, but only if the carrier of the modified DNA is a woman (since the heritability of mitochondrial DNA is strictly maternal). Moreover, the attempt to modify this type of DNA in the germ-line that has been reported was not done in order to achieve any special result regarding the features of the resulting child, but only to facilitate the successful procreation of couples burdened by very peculiar types of fertility problems. Nevertheless, however, it is in the report regarding the ongoing mapping of genetic traits relevant to athletic performance.

12 In conversation with various geneticists, I have been presented with the suggestion that genetic sequences inserted through gene therapy may be 'marked' in some way (such as a small part of 'empty' DNA of the type used for the so-called DNA-fingerprinting used in forensic medicine). Such marking may, it has then been proposed, be made obligatory through various regulations (such as rules for genetic research and for the patenting of genetic sequences) and subsequently used for distinguishing genetic variants which are present due to human intervention from those that are not. However, this suggestion presuposes that those who make use of gene therapy for enhancing athletic capacities will actually adhere to the requirements of such regulations – something that may be seriously doubted if such uses of gene therapy are covered by the ban on gene doping.

13 See Munthe (1999b) for a more in-depth argument to this effect.

14 To be more precise, cells that are neither part of this individual's initial cellular make-up, nor products of the regeneration of this make-up.

15 Edvard Smith, Professor of Molecular Genetic Medicine at the Karolinska Institute, made me aware of this important possibility. Professor Smith presented this idea at a Swedish conference on the use of genetic technology in sports – 'Sport, hälsa och genteknik' – held in Stockholm, 3 October 2002.

16 There are, it must be admitted, also the theoretical possibilities of the individual being a so-called genetic mosaic (i.e., carrying different genetic make-ups in different cells) and that this condition has been missed by the initial genome scan (which is not unlikely), or having been the subject of a local natural genetic mutation since the intial genome scan took place. However, the first of these conditions is extremely rare and, although natural mutations are not uncommon, the likelihood of any of these phenomena to be combined with a distinct enhancement of atheletic performance capacities is so unlikely that it may reasonably be claimed to be virtually non-existent.

17 Not that the picture needs any further complications, but it must be mentioned that this latter method may be counteracted if it becomes possible to turn the modified genes 'on' and 'off' at will, i.e., to intentionally and precisely regulate whether or not they produce any bodily substances that may be compared to the initial genetic make-up. In that case, athletes could have their modified genes 'turned off' up to the point of competition, eat or inject something (which may in itself be a completely innocent thing to consume) that turns them 'on' just before competition, and then again use the intake of something else to turn the modified genes 'off' as soon as the competition is finnished.

18 For a standard presentation of these issues, see, for example, 'Genetic Testing and Screening' in the *Encyclopedia of Bioethics*.

19 In particular, this concerns traits of relevance to athletic performance capacity, the heredity of which is more complex than classic monogenetic heredity.

20 See Radetzki *et al.* (2003) for more on this.

REFERENCES

Barritt, J.A., Brenner, C.A., Malter, H.E. and Cohen, J. (2001) 'Mitochondria in Human Offspring Derived from Ooplasmic Transplantation', *Human Reproduction*, 16(3): 513–16.

Encyclopedia of Bioethics (1995) 'Genetic Testing and Screening', revised edition, vol. 2, London: Simon & Schuster and Prentice Hall International.

International Olympic Committee (IOC), Official website of public documents, URL: Http://multimedia.olympic.org

Munthe, C. (2002) 'Prospects and Tensions in the Meeting of Bioethics and the Philosophy of Sports: Reply to Miah', in A. Miah, and S.B. Eassom (eds) *Sport Technology: History, Philosophy, Policy*. Amsterdam: JAI/Elsevier Science.

Munthe, C. (2000) 'Selected Champions: Making Winners in the Age of Genetic Technology', in C.M. Tamburrini and T. Tännsjö (eds) *Values in Sport: Elitism, Nationalism, Gender Equality and the Scientific Manufacture of Winners*. London: E & FN Spon.

Munthe, C. (1999a) *Pure Selection: The Ethics of Preimplantation Genetic Diagnosis and Choosing Children without Abortion*. Göteborg: Acta Universitatis Gothoburgensis.

Munthe, C. (1999b) 'Genetic Treatment and Preselection: Ethical Similarities and Differences', in A. Nordgren (ed.) *Gene Therapy and Ethics*. Uppsala: Acta Universitatis Upsaliensis.

Pérusse L., Rankinen, T., Rauramaa, R., Rivera, M.A., Wolfarth, B. and Bouchard, C. (2003) 'The Human Gene Map for Performance and Health-related Fitness Phenotypes: the 2002 Update', *Medicine and Science in Sports and Exercise*, 35(8): 1248–64.

Radetzki, M., Radetzki, M. and Juth, N. (2003) *Genes and Insurance*. Cambridge: Cambridge University Press.

World Anti Doping Agency (WADA) (2002) Official website, URL: Http://www.wada-ama.org.

10 Nutrigenomics, individualism and sports

Ruth Chadwick

INTRODUCTION

In considering the potential importance of the ever-faster developing field of genomics for sports, one might be tempted to think immediately of selecting for traits that are directly relevant to sporting performance. This possibility gives rise to a number of interesting philosophical issues, but they are not the subject of this discussion. Our genetic inheritance is, as we know, crucially dependent on environment. The drive to train budding young sportspersons from a very early age is testament to the importance of environmental influences. An enormously significant dimension to the range of environmental influence is diet. Indeed, one of the purported benefits of the setting up of large population databases such as the UK Biobank is to study gene–environment interactions including the interrelationship between genetic and dietary influences (see, for example, POST, 2002).

Even without the genetic developments we have seen in the past twenty years or so, it is no longer possible to exaggerate the importance of diet as an element in sports training. While the former England cricketer, Ian Botham, remarked in a recent interview that when he was in his prime as an international player, it was not uncommon to feast on hamburgers and a couple of pints, nowadays, diet is very carefully researched and controlled. Today, in the postgenome era, we are witnessing the entry of nutrigenomics into this field, as the importance of genes in human nutrition becomes increasingly clear.

First, some clarification is in order. To some extent the terms 'nutrigenetics' and 'nutrigenomics' tend to be used in ways that are not entirely distinct, but while nutrigenetics seeks to identify the minute individual differences, or single nucleotide polymorphisms (SNPs) that affect individual response to diet and which might affect dietary requirements, nutrigenomics, on the other hand, attempts to study the genome-wide influences of nutrition, to identify the genes influencing the risk of diet-related diseases, and to understand the associated mechanisms.

There are several possible applications of these developments. Nutrigenomics and nutrigenetics could have significant public health applications through understanding of how nutrition influences metabolic pathways; understanding of how this is disturbed in diet-related diseases; and understanding of how individual sensitizing genotypes contribute to such diseases. It has been suggested that nutrigenomics will seek to prevent the diseases that pharmacogenomics aims to cure.

In addition to the public health aspect, however, there are significant potential implications for individuals, and it is fair to say that until recently the ethical issues arising in relation to genetics and genomics have been addressed predominantly from the perspective of individualistic framings. Informed consent, for example, to sample donation; and access to and control of personal information, have been prominent in the field. As far as nutrigenetics is concerned, the prospects for individualised dietary advice, enabling consumers to adopt effective prevention strategies based on individualised prescriptions for their risk and susceptibility status *vis-à-vis* foods and food ingredients, prove exciting to a number of commentators, even though it is estimated that it will take several years to reach this point (Müller and Kersten, 2003). In the case of individualised diets, however, we have to consider not only prevention strategies but also the possibilities of enhancement.

What I want to argue is that, given the prevailing individualistic framing in ethics, and the role of the individual competitor in sports, we have to take seriously the possibility that a major driving force in nutrigenetics will be these possibilities of enhancement of performance through paying attention to such advice as nutrigenetics can offer. If this is the case, then questions arise as to how this will bear on sports ethics.

The significance of diet for the sports person was already long ago recognised by Aristotle, who used it in the *Nicomachean Ethics* as an example in his attempt to demonstrate his doctrine of the mean. The mean has to be determined not by seeking the average: what is right in one context may not be for another, just as the athlete has to eat quantities that would not be appropriate for the ordinary man:

> If ten pounds are too much for a particular person to eat and two too little, it does not follow that the trainer will order six pounds; for this is perhaps too much for the person who is to take it, or too little – too little for Milo, too much for the beginner in athletic exercises. The same is true of running and wrestling.

> (Aristotle, 1925: 1106a17)

Aristotle's point related to quantity: now the issue turns much more on the qualities of particular foodstuffs. Another difference in the present context is the recognition that dietary and nutrient requirements may need to take account not only of differences between occupational groups, but also of individual genetic susceptibilities.

As we consider the prospects of nutrigenomics and nutrigenetics for sport, however, a preliminary question is whether it is worthwhile. Is the effect of nutrigenomics really likely to be significant in terms of added value, over and above other kinds of nutritional research? There are concerns about its capacity to deliver on its apparent promises. One reason for doubt about this becomes clear when we consider the different between nutrigenomics and pharmacogenomics.

It might appear that there is a close analogy between pharmacogenomics and nutrigenomics. Pharmacogenomics, it is held, will enable drug prescribing on a much more individualised basis, and will be useful in reducing the incidence of adverse events (Housman and Ledley, 1998). Its promotion using the terminology of 'personal pills' is not insignificant: this again is attractive from the point of view of an individual-centred ethical perspective (Stix, 1998). As we noted above about diet, pharmacogenomic research should increasingly inform decisions both about quantity and quality: not only about the choice between drug A and drug B, but also concerning the appropriate dosage. So as far as this goes, then, it appears to be analogous to the promise of nutrigenomics to inform personalised advice about the appropriate quality and quantity of food. The relevant differences between the two contexts, however, are arguably greater than the similarities. Pharmaceutical compounds are very precisely characterised. They are also targeted at specific metabolic pathways. Food, on the other hand, is much more complex. Not only do foods tend to have a number of ingredients, but also specific nutrients can bind to multiple targets (Müller and Kersten, 2003). So in the sports context, in comparison to performance-enhancing drugs, it may be much more difficult to come up with sufficiently precise recommendations, and for that reason nutrigenomics and nutrigenetics may appear to be less attractive to sports participants.

Nevertheless, it is important to remember that the context of elite sports is one in which the tiniest of margins can make a difference to, for example, the breaking of a world record. If the purported sports-related application of nutrigenetics were that it would enable individuals to identify which nutrients would be likely to maximise their performance, even by miniscule amounts, it is not unlikely that it would prove attractive.

It is possible to see how this might work by exploring the example of using 'functional foods' in relation to sport. In fact, I would argue that the combination of nutrigenetics with functional foods may provide the primary example of the use of genetic information in sports for enhancement purposes. Functional foods are foods which have a specific health-promoting effect over and above their nutritional value (Chadwick *et al.*, 2003). They make a health claim, which may be related to prevention or enhancement. Examples that we already see on the market include cholesterol-lowering products and probiotic yoghurt. Functional foods might be of particular relevance in sport, however, as the following example shows. Let us consider the (not unlikely) possibility that a functional food, Supercon, were produced, claiming to have a specific effect that would be relevant to sport, such as improvement of concentration. There have been a number of ethical concerns associated with functional foods, arising partly from the fact that, being foods, they are tested for safety but not for efficacy, unlike drugs. We will assume, however, for present purposes that it does work and is not a 'con' in that sense. This might be relevant to any sportsperson, as arguably improved concentration is an 'all-purpose trait' where sports performance is concerned.

Furthermore, in the present context, such a functional food would presumably be regarded as preferable to the taking of a banned drug, which might have the same effect.

Being classified as foods, functional foods are placed in supermarkets alongside traditional products and yet they might not be suitable for all those who buy and consume them. The way in which they are advertised, however, is potentially misleading, for example, advertisements for cholesterol-lowering produces may use role models, who are apparently not in the high risk group for raised cholesterol, to eat the products in TV ads. As the range of products including particular ingredients increases, there are further concerns about overdosing. In light of the fact that the regulatory system approves these products on a case-by-case basis, there are clear difficulties about how to control the global effect on diet.

This is where nutrigenetics could be helpful in promoting informed choice about functional foods. Let us suppose that genetic variants A, B and C have been identified such that A responds 'normally' to Supercon, experiencing an increase in concentration of 10 per cent. People with variant B, however, have an adverse reaction to the functional ingredient, causing them to suffer an allergic reaction. People with variant C, on the other hand, improve their performance by 20 per cent, double the improvement experienced by group A.

This information would clearly be relevant to sportspersons considering the consumption of Supercon. It would enable variant B to avoid the functional food, variant A to benefit to a certain degree, and variant C to have the competitive edge as regards this characteristic. We could modify the example slightly, however, so that a similar functional food, 'Achieve', is put on the market by a rival food manufacturer. Although similar in effects, it has a slightly different configuration of ingredients, so that people with genetic variant B can take it and achieve an improvement in performance equivalent to that achieved by group C in taking Supercon. When we consider this modified example, it seems clear that it would be even more important to potential competitors to make their choice of functional food in the light of as much information as possible about the probability of beneficial and adverse reactions for people with their particular genetic make-up. From the perspective of individualistic ethics, this eventuality could be supported on the grounds of facilitating individual choice.

ETHICAL ISSUES

Supposing that nutrigenetics were to appear attractive in sports, what would be the associated ethical issues? Some are generic to other uses of genetic information: others are specific to the sports context.

Research

In so far as this is a branch of genetics, there are questions about the research that would be necessary in order to produce individual dietary recommendations. As in the case of pharmacogenomic research, it would be necessary to collect large numbers of blood samples to conduct association studies, in order to identify the SNPs that underlie differential response to specific nutrients. The ethical issues arising in relation to this kind of population-based genetic research are undergoing extensive debates in other contexts, and typically relate not only to consent to the taking of the blood sample, but also to storage of the relevant information, which would be necessary in order to track the response over time. Once the information was stored, there would inevitably be questions concerning who had access to it. This includes not only the issue of whether individual research participants should have access to feedback about their own genetic information, but also the extent to which the information would be coded or anonymous; and whether it might be accessible by third parties. This is important because in genetic research of this kind, once samples are collected and stored they are, in principle, capable of being mined for genetic information of other kinds. Much has been written about the potential for discrimination and I shall not add to that here apart from mentioning it as an issue. A further and possibly the most significant issue, however, concerns the extent to which the information obtained will be reliable and significant. There are general concerns about the statistical reliability and replicability of association studies (Ioannidis, 2003), but also there are worries about the potentially misleading character of the information acquired. For example, it may be the case that information about susceptibility is taken in a more deterministic way than is warranted.

In the absence of very precise, specific and reliable information, probabilistic information may be criticised on the grounds that its recommendations are either so general that they did not require nutrigenomic research, or that they are insufficiently supported by evidence – and these worries are pertinent to the nutrigenetics project as a whole. Nevertheless on its website the company Sciona, which offers individual advice, argues as follows:

> Small differences in your genes can influence how well your body metabolises foods, utilises nutrients and excretes damaging toxins, all of which can affect your general state of health. By finding out if you have any of these small variations, Body Benefits nutrition can provide you with specific dietary information that cannot be obtained from any other source.[1]

Enhancement

While the above claim relates to one's 'general state of health', in the sports context, what is most interesting is not health as such but enhancement. In genetics generally there has been a considerable amount of discussion about the conceptual and moral distinction between therapy and enhancement, and this is relevant both in medicine and in sports. While in the medical context, however, the therapy–enhancement distinction may be considered very significant (even if philosophically contested) because of the need to make tough public policy decisions about needs and allocation of resources, the sports context is overtly concerned with enhancement. Enhancement is in an important sense the goal, although we may want to distinguish between personal enhancement and enhancement of the general standard of performance in a given sport. The Council of Europe, for example, has recognised the pressures put on sport by 'the race for success, the need for stars' (Council of Europe, 1992). This point relates to ideas about the general nature and purpose of sport, an issue to which I shall return.

The point about personal enhancement draws our attention to the fact that sports persons have always used food in a 'functional' way. The passage in Aristotle's *Nicomachean Ethics* may be read as presupposing a function for food over and above nutrition. Eating to control hunger/maintain well being is not the main issue: eating to enhance performance is. The choice of food has become more precise in order to deliver particular results. This suggests that while functional foods raise issues for sports, conversely, the context of sport also raises questions about the concept of functional foods – namely, what is new in identifying certain foods today as 'functional'.

The concept of functional food is indeed not entirely clear. It may be helpful, however, to stipulate that functional foods, as I am using the term, are a subset of 'novel' foods – in other words they are foods that have not formed part of the normal diet of the population in question;[2] and they make a specific health-promoting claim, as noted above. Novel foods may be but need not be genetically modified (GM) foods, but although tomatoes, for example, contain lycopene, which is associated with a health-promoting effect, being an anti-oxidant, they are not a functional food in the relevant sense because they are not a novel food. Of course, tomatoes could be modified in such a way as to qualify as a novel food with a specific health-promoting effect and then they would be a functional food in the relevant sense.

Risks

Risks to individuals may arise either from the genetic test or from the intake of the food substance. As far as the risks of the genetic test are concerned, these arise not so much from the testing process as from the potential misuse of the information gained therefrom, as discussed above. Turning to the food itself, however, there may of course be concerns about safety and overdosing. A given food in itself might have deleterious effects as well as advantages. The idea of a food that is dangerous 'in itself', however, may be misleading. People have died or been hospitalised from overdosing on substances as apparently innocuous as carrot juice and even water. Indeed, it is here that precise genetic information might help to determine the risk to specific individuals arising from the intake of particular functional foods. Thus, nutrigenomics and nutrigenetics may increase, rather than decrease, safety, just as it is envisaged that pharmacogenomics and pharmacogenetics will reduce the incidence of adverse drug reactions.

Children

This point leads nicely to an issue that is situated in the area of overlap between generic and specific issues, and that concerns children. While there may be reasons to think that enabling adult sports persons to make informed choices about what to eat for enhancement purposes is desirable, things might look rather different with regard to children. Again, there are questions with regard to both the genetic aspect and the food aspect. There are ethical issues concerning the desirability of giving children genetic tests at all. While we may envisage a future in which everyone will have their genetic profile on a swipe card for multiple use, at present there are good reasons for the view that children should not be tested unless it is a necessary condition of ameliorative medical treatment. While I shall not rehearse these arguments here, enhancement for sports purposes would not come into this category. If, however, it came to be regarded as in children's interests to administer genetic tests routinely in order to establish potential allergic reactions to foods, then why not test for possible enhancement interventions as well? In such a case it would appear that it is not the genetic test itself that is an issue: the distinction between therapy and enhancement reappears.

If making food choices for children on the grounds of enhancement for sports training were found acceptable, there could nevertheless be a concern that parents eager to maximise their child's performance might be over-zealous in promoting the eating of a certain food, as they currently may be with regard to practising and training at the expense of other pursuits of childhood. The Council of Europe's Recommendation No. R (92) 14 on the code of sports ethics urges the recognition of 'the special requirements of the young and growing child' and an understanding of 'the biological and psychological changes associated with children maturation'. Furthermore, it is stated that the health, safety and welfare of the child or young athlete must be the first priority. While there may be cause for concern if over-enthusiasm for sports success worked against the provision of a balanced diet, there is no reason to suggest that either nutrigenetics or functional foods in themselves would produce this: the concern is not specific to this context.

ARGUMENTS SPECIFIC TO NUTRIGENOMICS AND SPORTS

Arguably, then, functional food is not an issue in itself, as long as it is a food. The difficult issues arise over when and where a functional food becomes a drug. For when the use of drugs counts as 'doping' in sport, there is a large body of opinion that this is incompatible with fair play (e.g., Council of Europe, 1992). There are different issues here: first, that functional foods may themselves be drugs; second, that food may be used as the vehicle for medication, as in the delivery of vaccines through bananas. In the present context, it is the former, and not the latter, that is at stake. Indeed, what I want to suggest is that the problematic issues arise not so much from the use of functional foods *per se*, nor from the informing of their use by nutrigenetics, but from the undermining of the boundary between food and drugs. The combination of nutrigenomics and functional foods has the potential to produce an increasing medicalisation of nutrition, which could lead to the reappearance of the 'doping' debate in a new guise.

As noted above, food and drugs are regulated differently, which reflects views about the essential differences between them. One purported difference is that while food is a necessary requirement of survival of the whole organism even in the absence of ill-health, pharmaceuticals contribute to survival in so far as they target specific processes when healthy functioning is damaged or at risk (Chadwick, 2000). In so far as the dividing line between food and drugs is undermined, we may need to revisit the ways in which at society level we deal with the conceptual and regulatory issues around the boundary between food and drugs, and the use of such foods in competition. As far as regulation is concerned, the regulatory regime for novel foods generally is already quite well established, but not in a way that is specific to competition.

The more subtle effects of the increasingly fuzzy boundary between drugs and food may concern our relationship with food, as our food choices become increasingly 'functional overall', over and above what we would most like to eat. I have suggested that nutrigenomics and nutrigenetics may foster the use of functional foods, but beyond that, even if foods do not fall into the category of functional foods as defined above, they are likely to reinforce a functional approach to food generally, so that objectives other than nutrition are sought. While this may be disadvantageous to those consuming them, it is not an inevitable consequence.

The question remains, however, as to the implications for sport, if it becomes increasingly difficult to distinguish foods from drugs. Perhaps the fuzzy boundary between foods and drugs will be more likely to change attitudes to drugs in sport, rather than the other way round.

Although the prevailing view is that the use of drugs to enhance performance is incompatible with fair play, this is by no means universally held (Edgar, 1998). Our assessment of it is related to our view of sport, and this will also be true of our view of nutrigenomics in sport. One view is that the purpose of sport is to promote self-understanding (ibid.). As Andrew Edgar has pointed out, this idea is under-theorized. Self-understanding has been held to be under challenge from the intrusion of genomics into design and selection (Habermas, 2003) of human beings, but nutrigenomics is a poor target for arguments of this kind. At one level, the greater understanding of the human genome and the underlying mechanisms of gene–diet interaction with regard to sporting performance should facilitate our self-understanding as biological beings with certain potential.

When we add drugs into this scenario, Edgar suggests that the objection to drugs presupposes that sport is a test of this innate biological capacity, which is disrupted by their use. On the other hand, if we suppose that sport is a test of character rather than biological ability, the objection is that drugs reduce the scope for effort. Edgar continues:

> if all athletes are taking drugs then, all other things being equal, the standards of the sport as a while will rise, and the mediocre athlete will have to work as hard as before to compete with the elite. What might, conceivably, turn out to be unequal, is the responsiveness of individual athletes to drugs.
>
> (Edgar, 1998, p. 223)

This is analogous to what is involved in nutrigenomics, if we substitute 'food' for 'drugs'. The mediocre might gain an advantage, if a competitor with genetic variant C, who is less talented than a competitor with variant A, obtains double the improvement of A in response to eating the functional food Supercon. Edgar concludes that whether this is construed as unfair or not depends on the extent to which the meaning of the sport itself remains the same. What exactly is being tested by a given sport, and to what extent might nutrigenomics be compatible with that?

Two things seem clear: first, nutrigenomics undermines the possibility of drawing a sharp distinction between biological and environmental interventions in the pursuit of enhancement. Second, the issues in this application of genomics knowledge cannot be resolved entirely from the perspective of individualistic ethics. Conceptual questions need to be resolved regarding the boundary between food and drugs, and the challenge of functional foods to the meaning of sport and associated issues about drugs in sport.

CONCLUSION

I have argued that in addition to exploring the issues concerning the use of gene technology to identify certain genes or genetic factors that might enable us to select future stars, it is also important to consider the potential of ongoing research in gene–diet interactions. Nutrigenomics and nutrigenetics might prove very attractive to sports persons, who have long used food in a functional way, over and above nutrition. The new category of 'functional foods' might prove especially attractive to adult competitors who want to make informed choices about their diet and its potential effects in enhancing performance. It is difficult to find any objections to these developments in themselves, provided that due regard is had to children's overall nutritional needs as part of the training process. The most problematic issue is the extent to which the use of nutrigenomic information and functional foods might be regarded as a new attempt to seek an unfair advantage as in doping, or whether, conversely, it will change attitudes to the doping debate.

ACKNOWLEDGEMENTS

The support of the Economic and Social Research Council (ESRC) is gratefully acknowledged. The work was part of the programme of the ESRC Research Centre for Economic and Social Aspects of Genomics.

NOTES

1 http://www.sciona.com/coresite/products/nutrition7.htm (accessed 2 September 2003).
2 The Regulation (EC) 258/97 of the European Parliament and of the Council, defines a novel food as a food which has no significant history of human consumption within the Community prior to May 1997.

REFERENCES

Aristotle (1925) *Nicomachean Ethics*, trans. Sir David Ross. London: Oxford University Press.
Chadwick, R. (2000) 'Natural, Novel, Nutritious: Towards a Philosophy of Food', *Proceedings of the Aristotelian Society*, 100: 193–208.
Chadwick, R. *et al.* (2003) *Functional Foods*. Heidelberg: Springer.
Council of Europe (1992) Recommendation No. R. (92) 14 REV of the Committee of Ministers to Member States on the Revised Code of Sports Ethics. Strassburg: European Union.
Edgar, A. (1998) 'Sports, Ethics of' in R. Chadwick (ed.), *Encyclopedia of Applied Ethics*, San Diego: Academic Press 207–23
Habermas, J. (2003) *The Future of Human Nature*. Cambridge: Polity Press.
Housman, D. and Ledley, F.D. (1998) 'Why Pharmacogenomics? Why Now?', *Nature Biotechnology*, 16: 492–3.
Müller, M. and Kersten, S. (2003) 'Nutrigenomics: Goals and Strategies', *Nature Reviews Genetics*, 4(4): 315–22.
Ioannidis, J.P.A. (2003) 'Genetic Associations in Large Versus Small Studies: An Empirical Assessment', *The Lancet*, 361(9357): 567–71
Parliamentary Office of Science and Technology (POST) (2002) 'The UK Biobank', Postnote 180.
Stix, G. (1998) 'Personal pills', *Scientific American*, 279(4): 10–11.

11 Compulsory genetic testing for APOE Epsilon 4 and boxing

Julian Savulescu

INTRODUCTION

Chronic traumatic brain injury occurs in approximately 20 per cent of professional boxers.[1] Boxers with brain injury have varying degrees of movement, intellectual, and/or behavioral impairments. 'Dementia pugilistica' is a form of severe dementia that resembles severe Parkinson's disease or Alzheimer's disease. Chronic traumatic brain injury has also been documented in American Football, ice hockey, rugby, horse racing and soccer. It has been believed that this results from repetitive concussive and subconsive blows to the head and in boxers, is related to the number and severity of exposures to punches.[2] Brain injury in boxers is related to the following factors:

- increased exposure (i.e., duration of career, age of retirement, total number of bouts);
- poor performance;
- increased sparring.[3]

However, one important recent study by Jordan and colleagues also found that the risk of brain injury was related to the presence of the apolipoprotein (APOE) gene.[4] There are three forms of the APOE gene: epsilon 2, 3, 4, which I will abbreviate to e2, e3, e4. This is a small single study (involving only thirty boxers) and the results are described by the authors as 'preliminary'. This study showed that:

- If a boxer had less than twelve professional bouts, there is significantly less brain damage.
- If a boxer had less than twelve professional bouts, genetics has little effect.
- If twelve or more professional bouts, significantly more of those with brain damage had APOE e4.

In addition to chronic traumatic brain injury, boxing is also associated with acute traumatic brain injury. In Victoria, Australia, three boxers have died from blows sustained in the ring since 1974, the latest, Ahmed Popal, dying in April 2001.[5]

In June 2001, the Victorian government introduced compulsory magnetic resonance image scans for boxers when they register as a professional and thence every three years.[6] The scans aim at picking up early brain damage that might be worsened during a fight. Three boxers were banned from professional boxing on the basis of these scans in twelve months.[7] The director of the Australian Academy of Boxing argued that such scans were necessary to protect boxers from 'promoters, trainers and their own ambition'.[8] However, the Australian Medical Association, as do many other associations of doctors, continues to call for boxing to be banned.[9]

Following the research of Jordan and colleagues linking APOE e4 to an increased likelihood of traumatic brain injury, the government in Victoria showed an interest in introducing a genetic test for APOE e4 as a precondition for professional boxing.[10] A doctor advising the Boxing Regulator stated that he would support the Professional Boxing and Martial Arts Board if it wanted to prevent those who tested gene positive from boxing.[11] This chapter will address the issue of whether or not genetic tests for APOE e4 should be made compulsory and whether only those who do not carry a copy of the APOE e4 should be allowed to box.

I will argue that a genetic test for APOE e4 should be made available but not compulsory. In the eventuality of a positive result, boxers should be informed of the available evidence relevant to the risks involved in boxing and should be entitled to continue their career as a boxer if they wish to do so. However, regular performance testing and brains scans should be required of all boxers, with possibly a greater frequency for those with the APOE e4 gene.

EVIDENCE IS NOT CONCLUSIVE THAT THE APOE E4 GENE IS ASSOCIATED WITH AN ELEVATED RISK OF BRAIN INJURY IN BOXERS

Relatively little research has been carried out on the relationship between APOE e4 gene and brain injury in boxers. The study described above is relatively small (involving only thirty boxers) and the results are described by the authors as 'preliminary'. Additionally, there is potential self-selection bias in the sample.

Other evidence supports the hypothesis that APOE e4 is associated with an increased risk of brain damage in boxing. This variant of the gene is associated with death and poor outcome following acute traumatic brain injury patients in neurosurgical units.[12, 13] Studies in mice have also related this variant of the gene to memory deficits and poor recovery from head injury. It has been suggested that APOE e4 plays an important role in neuronal repair and antioxidant activity.[14]

However, there is currently no definitive or conclusive evidence that the APOE e4 allele places a boxer at a higher risk of developing dementia. The evidence is weaker by orders of magnitude than, for example, the evidence linking smoking to lung cancer and other diseases. Genetics is only one factor which contributes to the risk of brain injury in boxers. Genetics may play a minor role compared to exposure to boxing – it was irrelevant if the boxer had less than twelve professional fights in this study. Reduction in exposure to boxing would have a greater impact on the incidence of brain injury than regulating entry according to genetic status.

THE CURRENT LEGAL CONTEXT

Professional boxing is arguably a form of employment. Introducing compulsory genetic tests for APOE e4 for those who wish to box and restriction of entry into boxing for those who result positive seems to conflict with the law relating to employment and disability discrimination in many countries such as the UK and Australia.

The Recommendations of the Human Genetics Advisory Commission

The Human Genetics Advisory Commission in the UK has examined the issue of genetic tests for employment purposes and has issued the following recommendations.

Recommendations of the Human Genetics Advisory Commission on the use of genetic tests and employment.[15]

1   An individual should not be required to take a genetic test for employment purposes.
2   An individual should not be required to disclose the results of a previous genetic test unless it affects their current ability to perform a job safely or their susceptibility to harm from doing a certain job.
3   Employers should offer a genetic test (where available) if it is known that a specific working environment or practice, while meeting health and safety requirements, might pose specific risks to individuals with particular genetic variations. For certain jobs where issues of public safety arise, an employer should be able to refuse to employ a person who refuses to take a relevant genetic test.
4   Any genetic test used for employment purposes must be subject to assured levels of accuracy and reliability, reflecting best practice (in accordance with the principles established by the Advisory Committee on Genetic Testing in its publications).

Compulsory genetic testing as a precondition of boxing would be the first mandated genetic test as a condition of employment. This would be a very important precedent. It may be argued that the introduction of such a test would be inconsistent with the recommendations of the Human Genetics Advisory Commission on the use of genetic tests for employment purposes.

Disability Discrimination Legislation

In both the United Kingdom and Australia, as in most countries, there is legislation preventing unfair discrimination. A Disability Discrimination Act in both countries prevents discrimination against people with disability on the grounds of disability. It is not clear whether the definition of 'disability' covers genetic status. If it does, these Acts would prevent discrimination on the basis of the genetic status.

EXCEPTIONS TO THE LEGISLATION

There are exceptions in the legislation. First, currently, the Ministry of Defence[16] in the United Kingdom uses a biochemical test to identify sickle cell carriers. This test is used in the selection process for employment of pilots. Sickle cell carriers may have a 'sickling crisis' if they fly at high altitudes resulting in their death and the plane crashing. For this reason, aspiring pilots who are sickle cell carriers may not be employed. Part of the justification for this restriction is to prevent harm to others from plane crashes. This is arguably a case in which genetic tests are used for employment purposes and employment restrictions have been enforced on the basis of the results of the test. The case of boxers, however, is different. The presence of APOE e4 does not make the boxer more likely to put other people's life and safety at risk.

Second, an employer or other body would be entitled to discriminate against a person who could not carry out the job or activity because of the disability. However, possession of the APOE e4 allele is unlikely to preclude a boxer from being able to box now, even though it may make that person less likely to be able to continue boxing in the future (i.e. it is a predictive test). Thus restriction of entry of an asymptomatic person with no evidence of pathology from boxing on the basis of a predictive genetic test may constitute unfair discrimination.

Because the case of the boxer with APOE e4 differs both from cases in which people with the gene variant represent a threat to other people's health and safety, and from cases in which a disability prevents the potential employee from carrying out the job, the two justifications that have so far been used for either enforcing genetic tests for employment purposes and for discriminating on the basis of the disability or of the genetic status are missing. Compulsory genetic testing for APOE e4 and consequent restrictions of boxing for boxers with APOE e4 gene seem to constitute a departure from the recommendations of the Human Genetics Advisory Commission on the use of genetic tests and employment and a breach of relevant legislation, e.g. the Disability Discrimination Act.

One may object that sometimes medical tests are made compulsory. Compulsory testing, although rare, does occasionally occur. For example, HIV testing prior to entry into Australia as a resident or testing for highly contagious diseases such as Lassa fever. However, the rationale for existing compulsory testing is prevention of direct harm to others. Testing for APOE e4 would clearly not prevent direct harm to others.

PRELIMINARY CONCLUSIONS

So far, I have brought two main arguments against the introduction of compulsory genetic testing for APOE e4 for boxing and consequent restrictions of entry into boxing. One is that the results of research are preliminary and not conclusive. Further research is necessary before any action should be taken at a policy level. The other argument is that compulsory testing and banning people from boxing would represent a radical departure from the current legal precedents relating to the employment.

One might object that the fact that a course of action represents a departure from the current legal provisions does not mean that that course of action is unethical. Maybe it is the legislation which is unethical. Moreover, while the evidence on the relationship between APOE e4 and brain injury in boxing is so far inconclusive, and this may be a good reason to promote research, before enforcing any restriction in boxing. But what should the governmental response be, if it were found that the APOE e4 were in fact responsible for a significant increase in head injury in boxers?

For the sake of the argument, I will now assume for argument's sake, that the studies reported at the beginning of this chapter were conclusive and that the presence of APOE e4 in boxers proved to significantly increase the risk of chronic traumatic brain injury in boxers. If it were proved that APOE e4 significantly increased the chance of developing dementia in boxers, should genetic tests for APOEe4 be made available? Should it be made compulsory? In case of a positive result, should the boxer be banned from boxing?

This chapter will show that even if it was clear that APOE e4 were responsible for increased risk of brain damage, and even if compulsory testing and discrimination did not violate existing legislation, still compulsory testing and restrictions of entry would not be advisable and should not be introduced. What should be introduced is voluntary testing and, for those who are positive, regular performance testing and brain scans.

ARGUMENTS IN SUPPORT OF MANDATORY TESTING AND RESTRICTION OF ENTRY INTO BOXING FOR BOXERS WITH APOE E4

The following arguments support the introduction of compulsory testing and restrictions of entry into boxing for boxers with APOE e4:

1 *Duty of beneficence/protection of participants.* If it is shown to be a reliable predictor of vulnerability to brain injury, mandatory testing would reduce the incidence of brain injury in boxers. The State has a duty of beneficence (to do good for people), Therefore, it is the State's responsibility to enforce testing and prevent those at risk from boxing. Such a policy would be good for those wishing to enter boxing themselves as well as their families, employers and those they care for.

2 *Autonomy.* I have argued elsewhere that autonomous judgements are based on the relevant information available. We cannot make an evaluative judgement between courses of action – in this case to box or not to box – as this requires knowledge of the facts relevant to the consequences of each option.[17, 18] Compulsory testing thus arguably enhances people's autonomy.

3 *Justice.* Compulsory testing and restriction of entry would plausibly reduce injury and thus reduce the cost to the community of health care and social support for chronic brain injury. Given that health resources are limited, distributive justice would speak in favour of compulsory testing and restriction of those who are gene positive.

ARGUMENTS AGAINST MANDATORY TESTING AND RESTRICTION OF ENTRY INTO BOXING FOR BOXERS WITH APOE E4

The following arguments may be brought against the introduction of compulsory testing and restrictions of entry into boxing for boxers with APOE e4:

1 *Duty of beneficence vs harms associated with genetic testing.* It is not clear that enforcing knowledge of one's genetic status actually benefits the person over-all. It is widely acknowledged that there are potential harms associated with genetic testing in general.[19] For example, compulsory testing would result in some people discovering that they have the APOE e4 allele. Those with two copies are at an eight-fold elevated risk of developing Alzheimer's disease. Thus, testing for APOE e4 to predict risk of brain injury from boxing is also *de facto* testing for risk of developing Alzheimer's disease in the absence of head trauma. Currently there are no proven effective interventions to prevent the onset of Alzheimer's disease. Genetic testing for Alzheimer's disease is not routinely offered and, if offered, would be offered on a purely voluntary basis. Discovering one has an increased risk of Alzheimer's disease (even if one does not box) could result in depression and anxiety.

2 *Mandatory testing and autonomy.* One view is that in order to be autonomous people should be maximally informed; from this point of view there is nothing like 'an autonomous choice to remain ignorant'. Where the risks for health are great, people should be informed. Then, maybe they might be allowed to choose. For example, cigarette smoking is potentially a very risky habit. The State enforces information on the risks associated with smoking by writing those risks in capital letters on the cigarette packet. Smokers are 'forced' to receive information. Their autonomy is thus enhanced. They are still free to smoke – at least in places where they do not harm others – but they are informed of the risks.

However, from another point of view, people may autonomously decide whether they want to receive some sorts of information or not. The State enforces a certain type of information – it enforces information on the risks associated with cigarette smoking. The correlate would be requiring boxers to know the risks of boxing, including boxing if you are APOE e4 positive. But the State does not enforce genetic testing to evaluate the risk that each individual has of developing lung cancer prior to allowing each individual citizen to buy cigarettes. While such tests are not yet available, it is possible that there is a genetic susceptibility to developing lung cancer if one smokes. Nonetheless, it is hard to imagine the State requiring smokers to submit to genetic testing even when a genetic test of susceptibility becomes available.

If we follow the same principles which seem to apply to other risky activities such as smoking, the State may enforce information on the risks associated with boxing, but should not enforce genetic tests for those who wish to box, in the same way as it does not enforce genetic tests for those wishing to smoke. The State should make individuals aware of the risks that are in general associated with the activity they wish to do, but not aware of the risks that they as individuals run

Moreover, whereas it is unclear whether mandatory information is a violation of autonomy or not, restriction of entry into boxing for those who have APOE e4, may uncontroversially be considered a violation of people's autonomy. Autonomy means self-rule or self-determination. Respect for an individual's own free and informed choices regarding his or her life is respect for his or her autonomy. Respect for autonomy is a key value in liberal societies. Restrictions on autonomy are generally accepted only for the sake of the protection of others, in liberal societies. A person should be entitled autonomously to accept the risks of boxing, once aware of the risks. It is important to remember that the person who is gene positive is not affected at the time of performance. He is only more likely to sustain injury if hit. It is strongly paternalistic to interfere in such choices. There are indeed restrictions on people's autonomy for the sake of their own welfare. The law on seat belts represents a restriction on people's autonomy mainly (but not exclusively) for the sake of their own welfare. However, in the case of seat belts, the interference is trivial and the benefit to the individual is significant (and is not merely a benefit for the individual, but arguably for the society as a whole through reduced costs of health care). The interference in the case of the boxer is first of all significant: it may frustrate a significant plan, ambition and employment opportunity. Second, the benefit that it would have for the individual is not accompanied by any great benefit for society as the laws on seat belts arguably provide. In conclusion, (1) mandatory information about one's own genetic status is not uncontroversially an enhancement of a person's autonomy; (2) restrictions on entry into boxing may be considered a violation of individual autonomy.

3   *Implications for insurance.* Those who discovered that they carried the APOE e4 allele would be required to disclose this to insurance companies prior to taking out life insurance, disability insurance or superannuation. Because of its associations with elevated risk of Alzheimer's disease and heart disease,[20] this may result in increased premiums in insurance. Keays describes the case

of one woman who was denied life insurance because she carried the Huntington disease gene. Huntington disease is an inherited form of dementia which starts around 40 to 50. She was asymptomatic at the time.[21]

4 *Implications for employment.* David Keays has also described a case of an 18-year-old man with a family history of Huntington disease who was at 50 per cent risk of having the Huntington disease allele. He was allegedly denied employment in a government service unless he had a genetic test to confirm whether or not he actually had the Huntington disease allele.[22] In a similar way, it is possible that some employers might require the result of testing for the APOE e4 allele and might deny employment on the basis of it. It is not clear whether this would be in breach of the Disability Discrimination Act.

5 *Stigmatisation.* It is well known that predictive genetic test results may result in the perception that a person is 'ill' even though the person is well at present. The person may sense that he or she is abnormal in some way and may irrationally focus on the possibility of impending disease. Others may perceive that person as 'ill' or 'genetically inferior' resulting in stigmatisation. This may result in social alienation and reduction in marriage changes.

6 *Family members.* Genetic test results have implications not only for the individual tested but also for other members of his or her family. The children and siblings of a person who has a copy of APOE e4 are also at risk of carrying the allele. This may cause psychological distress in them and may cause them to blame the person who was tested.

If effective interventions are developed to prevent the onset of Alzheimer's disease, this will place responsibilities on the person tested to inform his or her relatives of their risk of Alzheimer's disease and the interventions available to prevent it.

7 *Legal implications for the boxer.* If the genetic material is stored (as it usually is), this may have legal implications for the person tested. It is possible that it can be accessed for legal and forensic purposes. One man was convicted in Scotland of recklessly infecting his girlfriend with HIV on the basis of a genetic test performed as a part of a research project with a promise of confidentiality.[23]

8 *'Sending the wrong message'.* The introduction of compulsory genetic testing for boxing might be perceived as sending the wrong message that boxing is a safe activity, provided one has the correct genetic make-up. The major factor in developing brain injury from boxing is boxing, not genetics. Exposure to boxing is a much more potent risk factor than APOE e4 status and restriction of entry according to genetic status without reduction in exposure misrepresents the relative risks. Even those without APOE e4 can suffer brain injury. People may confuse a (relatively small) reduction in significant risk with removal of significant risk. This risks over-emphasising one (relatively minor) risk factor among many.

9 *Other social implications.* The introduction of mandatory genetic testing would be a precedent with significant social implications. One basic principle of

genetic testing to date has been that prior to any testing, counselling should be provided which is non-directive, ensuring that consent is as free as possible. Genetic tests, like other tests, are only performed on competent people after they have their free and informed consent. Compulsory genetic testing would not be 'free'.

Importantly, testing for the APOE e4 allele is a predictive test. Even if a boxer has two copies of the allele, this does not affect his ability to box now. He is currently well (assuming other tests are negative). This test predicts the risk of future harm. Regulatory authorities are quite right to prevent people from boxing who are at a serious risk of harm now, e.g. those with existing brain damage, haemophiliacs, people with fragile bones (osteogenesis imperfecta). But it would be a significant and new step to prevent people engaging in an activity which may result in harm in the future. If consistently applied, it would apply to many high risk activities such as mountaineering, off piste skiing and surf fishing.

10 *Justice.* Considerations made regarding point 9 bring us to discuss the issue of justice. Previously in this chapter, I argued that considerations of distributive justice may be brought in support of mandatory testing for APOE e4 and restriction of entry into boxing for positive people. Restriction of entry would reduce the social costs associated with boxing with APOE e4 (in the eventuality that APOE e4 were in fact associated with increased risk of brain injury in boxing). Here the benefit for society would compensate the frustration of individual autonomy. However, if this argument from distributive justice were accepted, this would have important social implications in terms of people's freedom to direct their life in many ways.

Many voluntary actions place an individual at risk and have a significantly greater public health burden than boxing, e.g. smoking. As we have seen before, the State currently informs people of the risks that in general are associated with cigarette smoking, but does not force people who wish to smoke to take tests to know the actual risk that they run in smoking. A recent study showed that smokers who have APOE e4 are significantly more likely to develop heart disease than smokers without APOE e4. If compulsory genetic testing were introduced as a condition for entry to boxing, consistency would require that all people wishing to smoke be tested for APOE e4 and only those who are negative be allowed to smoke. The public health benefits of restricting access to smoking would be greater than restricting access to boxing because vastly more people smoke.

This chapter has so far shown that there are arguments in support of mandatory genetic testing for APOE e4 for those who wish to box and restrictions of entry into boxing for those who have the APEO e4 allele. These arguments have to do with the State's duty of beneficence, with enhancement of people's autonomy and with justice. However, there are valid objections that may be moved against these arguments and further arguments against the mandatory genetic test and restrictions of entry into boxing. Having considered these arguments, this chapter discourages the adoption of restrictive measures of entry into boxing, as well as compulsory genetic testing for APOE e4.

CONCLUSION: EDUCATION AND PROVIDING VOLUNTARY TESTING

Occupational health and safety legislation requires that employers warn employees of risk. I suggest that this should include warning them of the relationship between APOE e4 and brain injury and the availability of genetic testing. Boxing authorities should exercise a duty of care to ensure that potential boxers are maximally informed of the risks of boxing. This includes health promotion documenting the existing evidence relating to risk factors for brain injury, in particular, exposure, and including the relationship between APOE e4 and brain injury (and development of Alzheimer's disease). Offering – or even strongly encouraging – genetic testing (with appropriate independent counselling) would also increase the chances that individuals better appreciate the risk which boxing presents.

Vigorous promotion of understanding of risk is consistent with societal practice in control of other actions which mainly involve self-harm (e.g., cigarette smoking); it is consistent with the duty of beneficence and with respect of individual autonomy, and also has a positive impact on society at large, as it is likely to minimise societal burden that boxers may represent without impinging on individual autonomy.

These are general points that pertain to genetics and to sport. When a subpopulation of individuals participating in a sport may be at increased risk of injury or adverse effect, the population should be informed of the risks to this population, and the availability of tests (genetic or otherwise) or identifying those at elevated risk. However, the mere existence of risk in a subgroup in the population should not mandate compulsory testing or restriction of entry if one is tested and turns out to be at increased risk.

To participate in life's activities according to risk, individual or general, would be a dangerous precedent. Many activities might be judged 'too risky'. We would run the risk of grossly constricting the range of activities available to people. Most people wish to avoid risk – there is an inherent human barrier to excess risk taking. We do not need laws to prevent participation in risky activities. And to do so would be thoroughly illiberal. In short, we should educate, not involuntarily test or restrict the freedom to choose what we do with our lives, including what risks we take.

I have not addressed the separate question of whether individuals who engage in risky activities should be compelled to internalise the costs of their behaviour. For example, whether they should be required to pay for their own health care. Some have argued that smokers and alcoholics should not be eligible for organ transplants because they are 'responsible' for their own ill health. Attributions of responsibility are notoriously difficult to make. Moreover, to begin to make relatively arbitrary decisions about who should pay the costs of their risky behaviour would be to go down a road of restricting fundamentally what kinds of lives people lead. While boxing may seem to some to be a relatively worthless activity, and even if it were, there are many other activities which entail significant risks that would soon be put aside if we were to regulate participation and life according to risk. Many of our greatest achievements have occurred in the face of very significant risk. Life is about living rationally with risk, not avoiding it.

NOTES

1   For the purposes of this chapter, I will refer only to professional boxing.
2   McCory, P. (2002) 'Boxing and the Brain', British Journal of Sports Medicine, 36: 2.
3   Jordan, B.D. (2000) 'Chronic Traumatic Brain Injury Associated with Boxing', Seminars in Neurology, 20(2): 179–85.
4   Jordan, B.D., Relkin, N.R., Ravdin, L.D., Jacobs, A.R., Bennett, A. and Gandy, S. (1997) 'Apolipoprotein E4 Associated with Chronic Traumatic Brain Injury in Boxing', Journal of the American Medical Association, 278(2): 136–40.
5   Giles T. (2002) 'Boxing Brain Scans', Herald Sun, 12 Feb; news section: 3.
6   Cauchi, S. and Foley, B. (2001) 'Boxer Brain Scans Insufficient, Says AMA', The Age, 28 May; news section: 4.
7   Spriggs, M. 'Compulsory Brain Scans and Genetic Tests for Boxers – Or Should Boxing be Banned?', Journal of Medical Ethics, forthcoming. Available at http://www.jmedethics. com, see Current Controversies.
8   Bachelard, M. and Kerin, J. (2001) 'Compulsory Brain Scans for Boxers', The Australian, 1 June; news section: 1.
9   See Giles, op. cit., Cauchi and Foley, op. cit., Bachelard and Kerin, op. cit.
10 Spriggs, op. cit., Giles, op. cit.; Robotham, J. (2001) 'Pro Boxers Face Going Down for the Gene Count', Sydney Morning Herald, 1 June; news section: 1.
11 Robotham, op. cit.
12 Teasdale, G., Nicol, J. and Murray, G. (1997) 'Association of Apolipoprotein E Polymorphism with Outcome after Head Injury', The Lancet 350: 1069–71.
13 Friedman, G., Froom, P., Sazbon, L., et al. (1999) 'Apolipoprotein E-epsilon 4 Genotype Predicts a Poor Outcome in Survivors of Traumatic Brain Injury', Neurology 52: 244–9.
14 McCory, op. cit.
15 HGAC, 'The Implications of Genetic Testing for Employment', June 1999, http://www.dti.gov.uk/hgac/
16 Ibid.
17 Robertson, R. and Savulescu, J. (2001) 'Is There a Case in Favour of Predictive Testing of Children?', Bioethics, 1526–49.
18 Savulescu, J. and Momeyer, R.W. (1997) 'Should Informed Consent Be Based on Rational Beliefs?', Journal of Medical Ethics, 23(5): 282–8.
19 For a description of these potential harms, see NHMRC, 'Ethical Aspects of Human Genetic Testing', www.health.gov.au/nhmrc/publications/pdf/e39.pdf
20 Humphries, S.E., Talmud, P.J., Hawe, E., Bolla, M., Day, I.N.M. and Miller, G.J. (2001) 'Apoliprotein E4 and Coronary Heart Disease in Middle-Aged Men Who Smoke: A Prospective Study', Lancet, 358: 115–19.
21 Keays, D. (2000) 'Genetic Testing and Insurance: When Is Discrimination Justified?', Monash Bioethics Review, 19: 79–88.
22 Button, V. (2000) 'Genetic testing: call for reform', The Age 21 July.
23 Savulescu, J. (2001) 'The Myth of Confidentiality, the Patient's Good and Public Health', Australian Medicine, 13(10): 11.

Part IV

Genetic technology and the ethos of sport

12 *Citius, Altius, Fortius ad Absurdum*

Biology, performance and sportsmanship in the twenty-first century

Lincoln Allison

This chapter is intended as a speculation on what might happen to the idea of 'sport' and the nature and popularity of sporting competition in the twenty-first century as a result of the impact of bio-technology. In the arguments which follow, the reader should bear in mind two thought experiments: first, that all attempts to regulate drugs and doping in sport are abandoned and, second, that we will increasingly be able to 'build' athletes either by breeding them or by the insertion of genes into existing competitors, for example, to duplicate the effects of stamina-increasing drugs such as EPO.

The point of view from which I want to examine these issues relates to a tradition which I will provisionally call 'sportsmanship'. By this I mean a modernisation of the core values behind the re-invention of sport in the nineteenth-century English 'public school'. Although this re-invention originally occurred in a specifically English context, it had considerable resonance in other parts of the world – in the British Empire by imposition (to some degree), but also in France and the United States. On the other hand, it was far less influential in the modernisation of sport in Germany and the Soviet Union.

In its contemporary use 'sportsmanship' is now principally associated with the observation of a code of rules and norms that constrain performance and the desire to win. This meaning would be a necessary, but not sufficient, condition of what I am talking about; there is much more to it than that and perhaps I ought to refer to 'sportsmanism' to indicate the greater breadth. This sees sport as having two kinds of moral worth. Instrumentally, it is an important training – in many versions, the best training – in virtues which are themselves logically independent of the idea of sport. These include self-discipline, comradeship, co-operation and the capacity to deal with stress, among others. But sport also offers certain kinds of pleasurable experiences which are of great value. The narratives of risk and achievement in sport and the complex relation between mind and body give meaning to experience: sport offers what John Stuart Mill calls 'higher' pleasures[1] and what, more recently, Tibor Scitovsky calls 'cultural' pleasures,[2] though neither of these writers stresses the value of sport themselves.

Sportsmanism in this sense is to be contrasted with 'athleticism' which sees athletic performance and the improvement of human physical capacities as of intrinsic worth. The distinction is perfectly clear philosophically: to a sportsman a good game or race, conducted in a competitive but friendly spirit during which the competitors have experiences they will remember all their lives and, perhaps, smile when they remember, is something of value whether it involves good runners or players or poor ones. However, this distinction is almost never made politically: the case for sport is invariably put in terms of both physical excellence and sporting pleasures and virtues without any regard for the considerable degree of conflict between the two sets of values. This was true of the original enthusiasts for sport in the nineteenth century, but it remains true of current political debate about sport, whether the statements are made about it in the UK General Election of 2001[3] or the Swedish government's official sports policy. It is an interesting reflection, though, on cultural difference that the general noun for those who engage in sport in the English version of the English language is 'sportsmen' and 'sportswomen' whereas the American is 'athletes' (as in the NCAA's 'student-athletes'), a term reserved in England for those engaged in 'track and field'.

THE 'CITIUS' PARADOX

The founder of the modern Olympic movement, Baron Pierre de Coubertin revered the achievements of Dr Thomas Arnold, headmaster of Rugby School from 1828 to 1842 and counted *Tom Brown's Schooldays*, Thomas Hughes' fictional memoir of Arnold's Rugby as one of his favourite books. In the code and principles of the English public schools he saw the possibility of the revival of ancient values of prowess and chivalry which offered an alternative future to mankind to the models of commercial capitalism and bureaucratic socialism which seemed the dominant futures of his age. As with other anglophile French aristocrats like Alexis de Tocqueville and Hippolyte Taine, the discovery of the revival of values which might be thought of as aristocratic not in some backwater, but in the Anglophone countries, the epitome of modernity, was an exciting one.[4]

Yet the slogan of the Olympic movement became 'Citius, Altius, Fortius' – 'faster, higher, stronger'. In itself, this is an expression of what John Hoberman calls 'the performance principle', that there is value in physical performance as such. There is no doubt that Thomas Arnold detested such athleticism, especially the idea of athleticism attached to egotism and although De Coubertin was far from as obsessed by the idea of amateurism as some of the Anglophone sports administrators such as his successor, Avery Brundage, there seems little doubt that he would have been troubled by the sort of Olympic competition which took place between Ekkart Arbeit's East German creations and their Russian rivals.[5]

The confusion is one of means and ends. In the tradition of sportsmanism it is good to strive to be the highest or the fastest, but only as an expression of the human character and will and within an assumed and shared code of ethics which are the real aim of the striving. That aim is lost if the competition becomes one between technical solutions: one might as well have competition between horses or robots if what we really want is the fastest or the highest. Perhaps an analogy would be with education: it is good to strive to achieve high marks, but in the aggregate high marks are of no value. Wisdom and knowledge are the things that matter and high marks achieved by means which do not increase them are worthless or, perhaps, worse than worthless.

Differences between sportsmanism and athleticism

1   *'Intrinsic' value.* The idea that sporting performance has an intrinsic value is sometimes asserted, but more often assumed, within the tradition of athleticism, but it makes no sense within the tradition of the sportsman. Taken completely literally, the idea is absurd. Consider two arguments for its absurdity which I will call the 'Johnsonian' (in reference to Dr Samuel Johnson's category of activities of which one does not ask whether they were done well, but why they were done at all) and the Confucian.

The Johnsonian argument thus: when I was young I had a friend who could spit ('gob' in our dialect) across the Lancaster Canal. It was a remarkable feat; nobody else could even get close. But society gave it no value: there were no rewards and no institutionalised competition for excellent gobbers. Slightly more complex examples arise from the eating, drinking and face-pulling competitions (and even more bizarre examples of competition in other aspects of physical prowess) which are common among schoolboys and students. The 'value' of these achievements is only what we put upon them; in these cases it is fairly limited while, in the case of running and jumping, valuing the activity positively is far more common and more easily explained, though by no means universal and certainly does not follow logically from the nature of the activity. This is an argument which must be borne in mind in several contexts. It renders absurd, for instance, the idea of an equal or fair distribution of rights or opportunities to exploit one's talents since any concept of talent is a restrictive and arbitrary in relation to human activity.

The Confucian argument can be explained in terms of a Californian friend of mine (a triathlete, among other things) who has often chided me on the sedentary nature of many of the sports and games which are popular on British television, including cricket, bowls, snooker and darts. To which the obvious reply is that if what we admire in sport is really athleticism, we should not be watching human beings at all, but should spend our time at the dog and horse races. Humans are simply not very good at running and jumping, though horses are literally hopeless at snooker.

2   *Participation and admiration.* For the sportsman, participation, even at a 'low' level is the superior activity. In athleticism this is only true for the elite. Politically, the point of a sporting pyramid for athleticism is to produce its apex. The point of the apex for a sportsman is to suggest ideas and images: ends and means are reversed by the two outlooks. For athleticism, the quality of a contest determines its worth. For a sportsman, it is the drama: a 'selling

plate' won by a neck is better than a derby won by ten lengths and a village cricket match won off the last ball is better than Australia crushing England.

3   *Specialists and all-rounders.* Athleticism is the realm of the specialist; the highest achievement is to be really good, preferably the best, at one thing. A true sportsman plays many sports. I have remarked elsewhere that the decline of the 'amateur hegemony' was, naturally, the decline of the great all-rounder who could and did play many sports at a high level. There are many factors involved in this process, but the most brutally simple is that if you have a lucrative contract to play sport, the most frequent examples being in soccer, your employers are highly unlikely to allow you to compete in anything else which raises the risk of injury.

4   *Winning as the 'only' thing.* A great deal of nonsense has been said and written about the amateur tradition, meaning an absence of a will to win. Arguably, one might expect amateurs to have an even stronger will to win than professionals, sometimes fortified by a kind of moral righteousness in comparison to the time-serving careerism of those who do something for a living. But this argument applies only within the arena of contest and we would expect sportsmen to be prepared to sacrifice much less outside the actual arena in order to achieve success. For example, as the chairman of a cricket club I face dilemmas as to whether to aspire to take the club to a higher level – at which many of the existing members would have to be replaced – or to maintain it at the existing level which is suitable for the members. This is never a dilemma on the field of play, but it does arise in team selection (given the existence of several different competitions and forms of the game) and in recruitment.

THE CURRENT STATE OF SPORTSMANISM AND ATHLETICISM

Clearly, sportsmanism, as I have defined it, has been in long-term historical decline in the context of globalisation and commercialisation. But it has also shown considerable resilience and areas of revival. There is no doubt that audiences for sport (to different degrees in different cultures) still judge sport partly in terms of sportsmanship and that certain sports such as golf and snooker which are able to present themselves as having maintained these traditions are able to attract audiences as a consequence. There are many new institutions which can be far more easily justified by the ideals of sportsmanism than by those of athleticism. These include such diverse activities as sporting tours (especially in Rugby Union and cricket) and mass marathon running. It is also the case that, though the difference between the two traditions is often fudged politically, it is also vigorously contested in some contexts such as the wide-ranging and intense debates about college sport in the United States.

But athleticism is clearly in a bad way, given public cynicism about doping and the presentation of that issue in terms of 'cheating'. Not only did the commercial revenues of track and field athletics drop by about 80 per cent in the 1990s from their peak in the 1980s, but in some respects participation has reached farcical levels. In county championships in the UK, the traditional bastion of the sport, a survey in 2003 showed that more than one in eight events had no competitors at all while 58 per cent had three or fewer; a senior men's discus event was won with a throw of 4 metres![6] Of course, this is partly an index showing merely that athletic traditions are changing: it has to be put in the context of a relatively healthy sport tradition in schools and aspects of running which have never had more competitors. But it certainly suggests that there is no guaranteed future for traditional performance-oriented athletics.

In other words, although sport has never been 'bigger' in the world, at least commercially and largely through the power of television, I am arguing that both the major traditions which have justified and interpreted it are in crisis. The triumph of sport over the past century may not be sustainable and there is both room and need for a vigorous debate about the future of sport in the light of the bio-technical challenge.

The (contested) future of sport

As a prolegomenon to the consideration of the future of sport, I think it is important to remark that the dichotomy I have set up between 'athleticism' and 'sportsmanism' is not a simple one and certainly not the simple one that is assumed by many sports journalists and administrators. I am not trying to imply that sportsmanism is about amateurism, virtue and traditional values and therefore regards any biological enhancement as 'cheating'. This would be in contrast to athleticism which is commercial, professional, specialised and unscrupulous.

In the first place it must be noted that the most commercially successful of sports in the global televised market – such as association football, tennis, cricket and golf – are not especially subject to biological improvement. Here I am agreeing with and inverting Sigmund Loland's 'vulnerability thesis' which stresses that the sports most vulnerable to such improvement are those which are most specialised;[7] they include those where stamina is paramount and blood doping, EPO and the 'EPO gene' can make a huge difference to performance such as cycling, cross-country skiing and middle- and long-distance running. They also include drugs where muscular development is the dominant feature and steroids or steroid-stimulants such as nandrolone are useful such as weight-lifting and the throwing and sprinting events in track and field athletics. The popular sports all involve a range of mental and physical skills, rendering biological improvement marginal. There are no drugs for tactics, judgement or even ball-control. This is not to say that drugs are of no benefit to, say, footballers and there have been persistent rumours in England about Italian clubs using EPO on a regular basis (which have been entirely reciprocated). Recent research on English football reveals very low levels of positive tests, 80 per cent of which involved 'recreational' drugs which could not enhance performance. Footballers have tested positive for both stamina and muscular drugs, either of which could improve aspects of performance. Recent research at Leicester University suggests that we should have the usual reservations about the effectiveness of testing, but we must also bear in mind that footballers are much more easily testable than individual competitors because they can be located so easily.[8]

Much of the debate about the 'vulnerable' sports takes place on false assumptions about their importance. Throwing and weight-lifting, for example, are neither popular participatory sports nor are they significantly commercial. Cycling and cross-country skiing are popular only in very limited parts of the globe; even track athletics is a relatively small and declining sport: in the USA, the most successful country in the sport, it does not rate in the top ten sports in terms of following. Swimming has almost no following in normal times. It is possible to imagine the great mainstream of sport flowing on into the twenty-first century without any of these components. The myth that they are in some sense major sports is a peculiar consequence of twentieth-century events which compounded nationalism with globalism and state policy with individual ambition to create a space in which it was a self-fulfilling truth that weight-lifting mattered. Given revelations about doping and given, also, the end of Cold War rivalries, we might expect that space to disappear. But that expectation is confounded by the persistent glamour (originally Gaelic for magic) of the Olympic Games which still draws our eyes to the spectacle of 'our' weight-lifter competing against others under the eyes of the global village. How long that glamour will last, given that I have argued that it is not well rooted in sporting traditions, is debatable and subject to the caution that magic is not the same stuff as logic.

It is also important to note that, from a sportsman's perspective, biological enhancement is neither so important nor so obviously cheating as the media commentary obsessed with high-level performance would imply. I (still) play both tennis and cricket within pyramid systems. These involve great discrepancies between competitors in terms of age, access to coaching and practice facilities and (in the case of tennis) both genders. What matters in setting up competition is not some sense of equal opportunity analogous to a concept of social justice, but the brute fact of roughly equal performance and therefore uncertainty of outcome. There would be no point in having a competition between people of the same age and gender if that were not – in the proper sense – competitive. Far better to have one in which 60-year-old men play 15-year-old girls of the same standard as themselves. Anybody who improves their performance, by whatever means, simply moves on up the pyramid to a higher level. The problem occurs only at the top and the assessment of its importance therefore depends on one's philosophy of sport. In any case, older competitors often take drugs in order to compete, mainly pain-killers, anti-inflammatories and anti-arthritic drugs and it would be absurd for a sportsman to condemn these practices.

We should also acknowledge the propriety of some sympathy with certain kinds of enhancement of performance by elite sportsman. Take the (hypothetical) case of a rugby player who has all the speed, skill and courage to make it to the top level, but whose build is simply too slight for that level. Coaches or fellow-players advise him that 'if he doesn't take it he won't make it' so he disappears to

California for one summer, re-emerging 15 kilos heavier and noticeably more thick-set. Five years later he is established in club and national sides which are at the peak of their sport: he has the life he dreamed of instead of being an also-ran. If it is the case that others got there by the same route, then surely we cannot blame him? And even if it isn't, there are at least some sense of fairness which would give him a right to remedy his natural physical defects.

Loland warns us that without vigorous debate on these issues, sport may 'degenerate and vanish'.[9] John Hoberman has commented that gene doping might succeed where other doping has failed in 'blowing away the whole fabric of high-level competitive sport'.[10] It follows from my previous arguments that my reaction to these apocalyptic scenarios is complex. I wouldn't have any great regrets about the disappearance or degeneration of the sort of 'high-level' sport which has no solid commercial foundation and I believe seriously major sport (defined by its commercial success) is threatened only in marginal ways while the bulk of participatory sport might even be enhanced by the change to come as the values of athleticism are undermined and those of sportsmanship revived. But there is a great deal of uncertainty, complicated by conceptual contest. Different cultures – and different people – understand 'sport' differently. I note, in this context, that the indigenous Scandinavian word for sport, 'idrott', has its origins in the notion of a 'mighty deed'. By contrast 'sport' in England has, historically, had connotations of amusement which has elements of risk and wager. Thus the Oxford undergraduates of a century ago who spent their lunch hour betting on the kind of hat which would next pass the High Street bus stop considered themselves to be engaged in sporting activity whereas they would not have thought of physical training as sport – though it might have been a preparation for sport. We simply don't know which senses and forms of sport are going to prevail in the current situation of philosophical contest and technological possibility, but we can, at least, try to clarify the alternatives.

Twenty-first-century sporting scenarios

Consider the following five models of the future development of sport:

1   *Muddle on* as before. In other words, continue the presentation of sport as a broad church which is simultaneously a noble calling, one of the forms of extreme human achievement, a commercial business and, for most people, a hobby. The amount of hypocrisy required would be considerable, but that has been the amount of hypocrisy demonstrated so far. The kind of magical fudging of issues which surrounds the Olympic Games and other major international events might be the best resource for muddling on. Official claims about the much enhanced policing and enforcement capacities following the establishment of the World Anti-Doping Agency (WADA) in 1999 might also help, but it may be that already that battle is irretrievably lost. It was noticeable that during the discussion of research on doping in football in 2003 in England virtually every official spokesman for the sport referred to (track

and field) athletics as existing in a condemned cell which football must not enter. One possible scenario is that reputation turns, if at all, like an oil tanker and that a much cleaned-up sport could retain a dirty reputation for a long time.

2   *Gladiatorialism triumphant* in which the 'performance principle' becomes mass entertainment. Performers are a separate breed, sometimes even literally, no longer linked to the grass roots of their sport and no longer part of its culture and community. We sit back and admire the 3-minute miler and the 200-kilo rugby player who can run 100 metres in under 10 seconds.

The unknown factor here is how much of a market there will be for physical freaks as opposed to heroes. The thesis of the 'civilising process' in sport might suggest that such interest might decline as there have been declines in violent sports and in the use of human freaks in circuses.

In this scenario amateur sport could revert to being a set of hobbies and cults.

3   *Commercialism destroys athleticism.* The market turns out to be more supportive of the 'non-vulnerable' sports, those in which acquired skills and tactical knowledge are at a premium. Athleticism becomes a minority cult (much as body-building is now).

4   *Schism.* Just as it seems natural to refer to sport as a 'broad church', we must also consider another possibility drawn from religious history in which two schools of thought about sport set up rival institutions, the purist and the gladiatorial, so to speak. There have, of course, been such schisms in individual sports on many occasions and the idea of two rival Olympic Games is a remote possibility.

5   *The revival of amateurism.* I am not here referring to the technical and risible form of amateurism associated with the Olympic Movement under Avery Brundage or the Rugby Football Union before 1995, which was obsessed with the mere absence of payment, but of the principle that sport should be played primarily for the love of it with an emphasis on participation and the development of all-rounders.

These models are not exclusive; rather, they emphasise different possibilities, many of which are compatible. The question would be of the relative power of different tendencies rather than whether they would happen at all. All these processes are already happening. We are muddling on; gladiatorialism does seem triumphant in some spheres, particularly in the American major leagues and especially in the National Football League. The 'non-vulnerable' sports are thriving at the expense of the 'vulnerable' and new 'alternative' sports, often with an emphasis on participation and the rejection of elite sport, and amateur values remain resilient. Recent Danish evidence, for example, shows a marked decline in the watching of sport and an almost equal increase in participation over the past fifteen years (around 20 per \cent in each case);[11] this may be a general European tendency, though the figures are difficult to interpret and we would not expect the tendency to manifest itself in the same way in those countries whose football leagues attract the elite players and produce teams capable of competing at the highest levels of

European competition. In the context of bio-technical developments in sport there are many possible winners and losers.

NOTES

1   John Stuart Mill, 'Bentham', in Mary Warnock (ed.), *Utilitarianism* (Glasgow: Collins), 1962, pp. 78–125. Originally in the *London and Westminster Review*, August 1838.
2   Tibor Scitovsky, *The Joyless Economy: An Inquiry into Human Satisfaction and Consumer Dissatisfaction* (Oxford: Oxford University Press), 1976.
3   See the documents of the 'Sports Project' of the Performance and Innovation Unit (PIU) of the UK Cabinet Office on www.cabinet-office.gov.uk/innovation/ and the aims and objectives of Sport England on www.sportengland.org/about/about_1.htm. The author also looked at the election statements representatives of a variety of organisations made to the sports supplement of the *Daily Telegraph*, including Kate Hoey (Labour Party), Peter Ainsworth (Conservative Party), Menzies Campbell (Liberal Democrat Party), Adam Crozier (Football Association), Tim Lamb (English Cricket Board), Simon Clegg (British Olympic Committee) and David Oxley (Central Council for Physical Recreation). For Sweden, see 'A Swedish Sports Policy for the 21st Century' on www.regeringen.se
4   For a fuller account of this historical period, see Lincoln Allison, *Amateurism in Sport: An Analysis and a Defence* (London: Frank Cass), 2001, pp. 17–48.
5   For the controversy about Denise Lewis, the Olympic heptathlon champion in 2000, employing Arbeit as her coach see, for example, Sue Mott, 'Architect of Abuse who Coaches for Britain', *Daily Telegraph*, 3 May 2003, pp. S.4–5 and Michael Johnson, 'Lewis Has Acted Stupidly', *Daily Telegraph*, 9 May 2003, p. S.1.
6   Duncan Mackay, 'Britain Runs Low on Athletes', *The Guardian*, 29 May 2003, quoting material originally in *Athletics Weekly*.
7   Sigmund Loland, 'Technology in Sport: Three Ideal-Typical Views and their Implications', *European Journal of Sport Science*, 2(1), February 2002.
8   Research by Ivan Waddington *et al.* of the Centre for Research into Sport and Society at the University of Leicester, as first presented on *The Real Story* on BBC1 TV and on Radio 5 Live on 19 May 2003.
9   Loland, op. cit., 'Concluding Remarks'.
10 In an email to the author.
11 See Soren Schulz Jorgensen, 'Industry or Independence? Survey of the Scandinavian Sports Press', at www.play-the-game.org

13 The vulnerability thesis and use of bio-medical technology in sport

Sigmund Loland

INTRODUCTION

The use of performance-enhancing bio-medical technology in sport, with the paradigmatic example in what is usually referred to as doping, can be discussed from many angles. In the public discourse and the mass media, such use is often portrayed as a matter of individual choice and, in the case of banned substances, of individual shortcomings and moral failure. In the academic discourse we find more reflective insights. John Hoberman (1992) has written on the history of the use of performance-enhancing drugs, medical sociologists such as Ivan Waddington (2000) see drug use in the background of what is called the medicalization processes of society, and cultural critics understand excessive use of performance-enhancing technologies as expressions of a culture obsessed with unlimited growth and progress – a culture out of control (Loland, 2001b). In the literature on sport ethics, performance-enhancing technologies are discussed with reference to what is seen as 'the nature of sport', to fairness and justice, and to the health and well-being of athletes (Butcher and Schneider, 2000). All these perspectives, perhaps with the exception of the first, add significant insights to the field.

My approach here, however, will be somewhat different. The thesis will be that, in the quest for improved sport performances, the use of bio-medical technologies becomes morally problematic due to systemic characteristics of sport itself. More specifically, after some background comments, I will present what I call the vulnerability thesis and argue that sports with highly specialized demands on performance are particularly vulnerable to excessive use of bio-medical technology.[1] In the concluding section, I sketch possible implications of this view for future strategies in the dealing with bio-medical technology in sport.

THE TOTALIZATION PROCESS AND ATHLETES' AUTONOMY

A traditional sport ideal that is still valid, I think, is that sport deals with the quest for human excellence. Sport performances are admired as products of individual and team talent and hard and long effort from the very first training session until the very moment of performance in competition. The social organization of sport competitions reflects the idea that, at least to a certain extent, athletes and teams are given insight in, control over and responsibility for their performances. For instance, competitions are organized around the ideal of quality of opportunity to perform. To a great extent, inequalities with impact on performance over which athletes have little control and influence, and for which they therefore cannot be claimed to be responsible, are eliminated or compensated for (Loland, 2002). I am talking now of inequalities in external conditions, in weight, height, gender and age (classification), and in technology and equipment (standardization).

In the past couple of decades, this ideal has been significantly challenged by what the Finnish sociologist Kalevi Heinilä (1982) describes as the totalization process in international sport. As the political and commercial significance of sport success has increased, competitions have turned into struggles between total systems of human, economical, technological and scientific resources. The image of athletes competing against each other conceals the true picture. Heinilä talks of a 'hidden validity'. What is being measured in international sport is not primarily individual athletic skills but system strength.

One part of the totalization process is the development and increased significance of performance-enhancing technologies. Among these, bio-medical technologies seem to be the most powerful ones. I am talking now about everything from scientifically regulated training and diet programmes and nutritional supplements to the use of drugs and, in the future, genetic technologies. These are also the most controversial kind of technology in sport. One key characteristic is that they do not really require athlete insight and effort but depend almost totally for their efficiency on external expertise (Loland, 2001a).

The increased significance of expert-administered technology can be seen as problematic for many reasons. Some see it as opposing what they take to be 'the nature and essence' of sport, and some see it as unfair and unjust. Independent of one's normative sport views, however, it can be argued that when, in any human practice, insight in, control over and responsibility for conduct move from the individual to external expert systems, moral problems arise. What is at stake here is individual autonomy and the risk of individuals being treated as a means towards system ends.

In most sport communities, there is concern for the vulnerability of individual athletes in this respect. This is illustrated by, among other things, the ban on drugs and testing for and penalizing drug use. However, as indicated in the Introduction, the anti-doping campaigns are usually built on conceptions of immorality in individuals and sport groups and less on systemic insights into sport itself. This chapter is an attempt to complement our understanding of the use of performance-enhancing bio-medical technology in this respect.

ATHLETIC PERFORMANCE

My thesis will be that highly specialized demands on performance represents a systemic problem in sport as specialized performances are highly vulnerable to excessive use of bio-medical technology. To describe more accurately and justify this thesis, there is need for a more general understanding of what athletic performances are about.

An athletic performance is the complex result of a great number of genetic and non-genetic influences. The full story starts at the very moment of conception, and runs via influences from the very first nurture and biological and social-psychological environment, the physical, biological, psychological, social and cultural environment during childhood and youth, through sport-specific influences from the very first time at play and the first training session to the final preparation before competition, and ends in situational aspects of the actual competition and the moment of performance itself. To be able to critically discuss the use of bio-medical technology, however, it is necessary to make some analytic distinctions. One basic distinction, often drawn within exercise science, is between genetically programmed basic abilities, and learned skills (Martin, 1991).

Basic abilities can be grouped in to bio-motor and mental abilities (Bompa, 1994). Bio-motor abilities include strength, endurance, flexibility, speed and coordination. Mental abilities refer to sensation, motivation, emotion, cognition, and personality characteristics. Basic abilities are genetically programmed in the sense that, provided there are no genetic or serious environmental disturbances, they develop universally in all human beings. A certain level of development here is necessary for normal human functioning.

Different from abilities, skills are not genetically programmed in the sense that they develop universally – they must be learned in interaction with particular environments. Skills can be of general and specific kinds (Bompa, 1994). For instance, common motor skills in our society include walking in traffic, conduct in lines of various kinds, eating in socially accepted ways, and so forth. Specific skills are related to particular practices such as sport, where they are more or less defined in the norms and rules. In sport, it is common to distinguish between technical (motor) and tactical (cognitive) skills. A rule for technical skill in tennis might be 'Look at the ball when you hit it!' A rule for tactical skills in soccer might be 'When the opposing team is superior, play defensively and concentrate on breakdowns and quick turnovers!'

SPECIALIZATION

In a sense, all athletic performances represent specialization of a kind. The sprinter specializes in running the 100-metre as fast as possible, the soccer player specializes in playing soccer, or perhaps in certain roles on a soccer team, the decathlon participant specializes in the ten events that make up the decathlon. However, based on the distinction between abilities and skills, it is possible to discuss degrees of specialization between various performances.

The significance of various abilities and skills varies greatly between sports. Without a well-adapted nervous system and a high percentage of fast twitch muscle fibres, a track and field sprinter will have problems succeeding at a top level. As Sir Roger Bannister (1997) says, 'the faculty of speed is inborn'. Performance in sports with more complex technical and tactical requirements depends to a lesser degree on one-sided advantageous predispositions for the development of abilities. For instance, one soccer player might be a little slow whereas another has great speed. Both players can become top performers. The slower player might have excellent working capacity and tactical skills, the faster player might compensate for a certain lack of working capacity with speed and strong technical skills.

In other words, some sports, such as the running events in track and field, tend to narrow definitions of performance in a particularly radical way. Whereas playing soccer, or competing in the decathlon, is based primarily on learned skills, the successful Olympic 100-metre performance depends upon a fortunate genetic predisposition for, and a systematic and extensive development of, the bio-motor ability of speed. A more specific definition of specialized performances is that these are performances that are based primarily on one or two bio-motor abilities.

THE VULNERABILITY THESIS

Now specialized performances can be related to the use of performance-enhancing bio-medical technology. Bio-motor abilities are genetically programmed. This programming can be mapped in the genome; the total set of genes in the nucleus of a cell. Genes are codes for the production of various enzymes (catalysts of bio-chemical processes) and structural proteins, which are the building blocks of cells and tissues and the basis for development of bio-motor abilities. Hence, such abilities can be manipulated by bio-chemical substances and more or less advanced bio-medical technology. This provides a basis for the formulation of what I have called the vulnerability thesis:

For any athletic performance it follows that the stronger degree of specialization (the higher significance of basic bio-motor qualities and the lesser significance of technical and tactical skills in performance), the more vulnerable a performance becomes to bio-medical and bio-technological manipulation.

Let me take a few examples. A good sprint performance in track and field relies heavily on the ability to develop speed. Speed is based on reaction time, explosive strength, and efficient running technique. This integrated capacity for speed is to a large extent a development of genetic predispositions that can be manipulated in various ways. It suffices to point to the efficiency of anabolic steroids and, perhaps in the future, genetic technology to improve explosive strength. Therefore, sprint running is a vulnerable sport.

The sprinter's main tactical rule is simple. Their challenge is full speed from start to finish! Other running events in track and field, such as the 10,000 metre, include a stronger tactical element. In long races, athletes have to spread their energy optimally during the race. However, here endurance is a critical bio-motor quality, and endurance can be efficiently enhanced with, for instance, EPO (erythropoietin) that stimulates the production of red blood cells and enhances the capacity for oxygen transport.

The vulnerability thesis does not primarily distinguish between sport events but between various forms of sport performances. American Football can serve an example of a sport that includes both vulnerable and less vulnerable performance requirements. This is a complex sport but with specialized role requirements. A defender has to be strong in mass velocity, which again is based primarily on the bio-motor abilities of speed and strength. A running back depends upon speed although the skills of tactical running and catching the ball are important. Both the defender and the running back can improve significantly through the technological enhancement of explosive strength. A quarterback needs good technique, good tactical understanding of the game and good all round bio-motor skills. The use of steroids will be of less significance. This is the position that requires the most complex skills and that has the lowest degree of vulnerability.

European football and tennis are built on less specialized performances and are therefore less vulnerable. These sports require complex technical and tactical skills. There are no pills or injections that can significantly enhance technical and tactical skills. Of course, favourable genetic predispositions for the development of various abilities are important, but good players need an all-round profile in order to learn the skills necessary to succeed. And skills are learned through extensive practice, primarily in social interactions. In both sports we find elite players with a diversity of talent, abilities and skills.

CONCLUSION

I have argued that the use of bio-medical technology to enhance performance is more relevant in sports with specialized performance requirements than in other sports. In light of the possibilities of great pay-offs in sport success, specialized performances are considered vulnerable to excessive use of such technology. The moral problem involved is that individuals easily become mere means towards the realization of system interests. In vulnerable sports in particular, athletes can end up as guinea pigs, or as uninformed and irrational agents, in grand expert-administered experiments on their own performance capacities. The possible consequences of the systematic affinity of specialized performances to excessive use of bio-medical technology are manifold. Let me conclude by pointing to what to me seems to be the most important ones.

If my argument holds water, traditional anti-doping strategies built on ideas of individual and group responsibilities might seem reactive strategies. One might deter athletes from using drugs for a while, but gradually such use will develop and become wide-spread as part of the systemic 'logic' of sport, so to speak. Traditional anti-doping work does not satisfactorily address these systemic problems and the chances for success might seem grim.

The vulnerability thesis can give rise to more constructive strategies. A pro-active approach could aim at systemic changes in sport itself. Elsewhere, and with track and field as my practical example, I have explored such action in more detail (Loland, 2001b). I have argued that specialized performances represents a small-scale version of the ecological crisis, and that alternative schemes of development can be inspired by the ecological ideal of sustainable development, in particular, ideals of diversity and complexity. In diverse and complex sport cultures, performances are the products of complex interactions of bio-motor abilities and technical and tactical skills, and individuals have a high number of potential ways of realizing their talents and interest.

To some, these ideas might seem utopian. Some of the most specialized performance sports, such as the 100-metre sprint in athletics, are among the most popular media events on the international entertainment market. They give rise to immense pay-offs in terms of profit and prestige. We should be under no illusions about the willingness to systemic changes in what today seems to be a winning formula.

At the same time, however, the idea of less vulnerable sports may not be as utopian as it may seem. The preferences of the sport public can change within shorter frames of time than one might expect. In fact, I think that there are clear signs of a development towards less vulnerable sports already. Technical and tactical complexity, characteristic of less vulnerable sports, belongs to the world of sporting games, such as soccer, basketball, and volleyball that actually are the most popular sports in terms of public attention. Moreover, new sports with new ideas of progress and growth are appearing on the scene. The so-called board sports – surfing, skate boarding, snow boarding, wake boarding, and kite boarding – are good examples. With their relatively non-precise measurements of technically (and tactically) complex performances, and with their lack of well-defined, standardized conditions, they might become a less vulnerable performance paradigm in times to come.

NOTE

1 This chapter, in particular the sections about athletic performance, specialization, and the vulnerability thesis, is built on my 'The Vulnerability Thesis and its Consequences – A Critique of Specialization in Olympic Sport', to be published in an upcoming collection of essays (edited by John Bale and Mette Krogh Christensen) on Olympic sport.

REFERENCES

Bannister, R. (1997) 'Human Performance in Athletics: Scientific Aspects of Record Breaking', paper presented at the IAF seminar, 'Human Performance in Athletics: Limits and Possibilities', Budapest, Hungary, 11–12 October.

Bompa, T.O. (1994) *Theory and Methodology of Training. The Key to Athletic Performance.* 3rd edn. Iowa: Kendall/Hunt.

Butcher, R.B. and Schneider, A.J. (2000) 'A Philosophical Overview of the Arguments on Banning Doping in Sport', in T. Tännsjö and C.M. Tamburrini, (eds) *Values in Sport*, London: E & FN Spon, pp. 185–99.

Heinilä, K. (1982) 'The Totalization Process in International Sport', *Sportwissenschaft*, 2: 235–54.

Hoberman, J.M. (1992) *Mortal Engines: The Science of Performance and the Dehumanization of Sports*. New York: Free Press.

Loland, S. (2001a) 'Technology in Sport: Three Ideal-Typical Views and Their Implications', *European Journal of Sport Sciences*, 2, 1. Available at http://www.tandf.co.uk/journals/titles/17461391.asp

Loland, S. (2001b) 'Record Sports: an Ecological Critique and a Reconstruction', *Journal of the Philosophy of Sport*, XXVIII: 127–39.

Loland, S. (2002) *Fair Play: A Moral Norm System*. London: Routledge.

Martin, D. (ed.) (1991) *Handbuch Trainingslehre*. Schorndorf: Hofman.

Waddington, I. (2000) *Sport, Health, and Drugs*. London: E & FN Spon.

14 Sport, gene doping and ethics

Gunnar Breivik

INTRODUCTION

On 11 May 2001, Jere Longman wrote an article in *The New York Times* where he raised a series of questions that triggered a debate in both International Olympic (IOC) and the World Anti-Doping Association (WADA). He asked whether it would be possible in the future to inject a gene that could result in more fast-twitch muscle fibres, enabling a sprinter to run 100 metres in 6 seconds instead of just under 10. And could one in a similar way inject a gene that increases the oxygen-carrying capacity so that a marathoner could run 26.2 miles in one and a half hours instead of just over two? Some believe that such a development lies far ahead in the future. Others believe injections are only a few years away. And still others think that we already have gene doping in elite sports today.

We do not know how fast new genetic techniques will develop and how they will influence the development of future sport, but we should not underestimate the problems. The human genome has been mapped; cloning of animals is a fact. In November 2001 the first human embryo was cloned by the American company Advanced Cell Technology. Gene therapy as treatment for various health defects and illnesses is under way.

The development of new genetic techniques raises questions that will affect future elite sport. The top sprinter Maurice Greene is one of many who ask whether manipulation of an egg or embryo should be considered cheating. If an elite athlete is produced in that way, it is not the athlete himself who has done something wrong. Should athletes of this kind automatically be disqualified for participation in Olympic Games? On which grounds?

In this chapter I will discuss problems that surface in the aftermath of the new genetic techniques. I shall first describe some central aspects of the ideological foundation of modern elite sports. The point is to show that doping is a natural consequence of the development of elite sport and not an accidental aspect of it. I shall then, in the next part, look at traditional doping, see how doping has been defined and the ethical problems that doping has raised. In the third section I shall sketch the new genetic techniques and the new ethical problems they create. Finally, I will discuss whether and how the genetic technology challenges the idea of sport and sport competitions. What does it mean to be an athlete? What do we measure in sport competitions? What is the outcome? What are the implications of elite sport for human identity, autonomy and dignity?

THE IDEOLOGICAL BASIS OF MODERN ELITE SPORT

Doping has followed elite sport right from its start, both in antiquity and in modern times (Prokop, 1970). Doping is therefore not an accidental trait of elite sport but rather a natural consequence of it. Elite sport is increasingly characterized by the pursuit of advantages. Athletes want to have means that are efficient and that the other competitors do not (yet) have. Some of these means are legal, others are not. And some are in a legal and ethical grey zone. Several factors have contributed to the hunt for advantages and the development of new doping means. Let me mention three factors.

First, modern elite sport was for a long time considered to be a contrast to Greek sport with its weight on harmony between body and soul. According to newer research this is a myth that was developed in European upper-class circles in the middle of the nineteenth century (Young, 1984). Greek Olympic sport had a very strong focus on victory and success. To be defeated was considered a serious shame and damage. Greek sport was individualistic, often brutal, with use of doping, with huge money rewards, professional athletes, the cult of heroes and entertainment for the public. Modern elite sport has many parallels to Greek sport. But there are also differences, such as the belief in continuous progress and the pursuit of records. The idea of a systematic and continuous progress originated in the fifteenth century. It was further developed during the Enlightenment period to a theory of a global, technological progress by means of science and reason (Nisbet, 1980).

Modern elite sport is inextricably tied to the idea of progress. The Olympic motto 'citius, altius, fortius' – faster, higher, stronger – is perhaps the most concentrated expression of belief in eternal progress. To set records has been almost as important as winning (Guttmann, 1978). To break barriers, do the impossible, has followed modern elite sport all the time (100 metres in 10 seconds, one English mile in 4 minutes, pole-vault 6 metres, long jump 9 metres, and so on). The hunt for progress and records has been like a motor that has propelled the search for advantages of various kinds, including doping.

Second, liberalism as developed in the tradition of John Locke, contained the idea of a freedom marked with open access for actors who compete and are rewarded according to performance, in compliance with implicit and explicit rules (the invisible hand, personal moral, market regulations). Modern sport is the true child of liberalism. In principle, sport offers open access to actors to test their abilities against other actors under equal conditions, according to fair rules and with rewards according to achievements (Breivik, 1998). The liberal society is an achievement society. In many ways, sport is the perfect model for the achievement society. Nowhere else are the abilities and achievements of the actors tested in such an open, fair and direct way. The increasingly harder competition in elite sport and the extreme focus on winning and rewards have contributed to a more and more extreme hunt for advantages and to new forms of doping.

Third, the modern society and its development are increasingly based on scientific and technological development. Technology creates new possibilities, but also new dangers (Kemp, 1991). Modern elite sport is in many inextricable ways tied to the general technological development of modern society. But more important in this context is the intimate connection between technology and sport to increase human performance (Ravn and Hansen, 1994). Equipment and facilities are tailored to athletes with more extreme bodily abilities and better technical skills. Technology and research adjust and adapt the equipment until it is a direct continuation of the body and its parts (the ski, the bicycle, and the parachute). The surface and the forms of the body are manipulated with body building, body sculpturing, operations, and textiles. And even more, the inner organs and systems of the body are manipulated by diets, nutritional supplements, doping means. And we can add techniques of mental preparation and advanced systems of biofeedback. Behind this development we find a more comprehensive and systematic use of research. This coupling of sport with science and technology has followed modern elite sport right from its start (Hoberman, 1992). The continuous interest in scientific testing of the limits of human performance is part of the modern idea of elite sport (International Athletic Foundation, 1997).

The pursuit of records, the importance of winning, the use of new technology, are central background factors of modern elite sport that have also been instrumental in the coupling of elite sport with doping. In addition, there are several social and cultural factors. East Germany set up a system of doping in order to have success in international elite sport and thereby promote the socialist political and economic system. In the capitalist world, sport has in a similar way been used as the showpiece for the country and its system. Media focus and public interest, commercialisation and sponsoring, professionalism and extreme achievements are all connected. Together they contribute to the more and more intense hunt for advantages and thereby propel the search for new and more advanced forms of doping (Tangen, 1997). The so-called 'limelight effect' implies that the winner takes all, media focus, status, prestige, money and popularity. When this is no longer limited to the single athlete but is enlarged to the team, the support system, the sponsors, the equipment producers, the public, then sport competitions become fights between systems that fight to win technological, commercial, and national 'battles' through sport (Breivik, 1998).

THE PROBLEM OF DEFINING DOPING

Doping comes from the South African Kaffir dialect where 'dop' is the word for a strong liquor (Prokop, 1970). Various forms of artificial stimulation have been used in different cultures to increase performance in war, work, games, and religious cults.

Doping has been defined in the different ways, depending on the context. In modern sport the key element in the various definitions of doping has been the notion of artificial improvement of performance. There have been several problems with such a general definition. What is 'artificial'? IOC therefore dropped the general definition and instead set up a list of substances and methods that were considered as doping means (Wilson and Derse, 2000). Administration of the list of prohibited substances and methods has now been taken over by WADA (2003). WADA first had the idea of setting up a list of substances and methods that could be shown to have a performance-enhancing effect. The substances and methods that had negative health effects, but no performance effects, should be dealt with through a medical list that should encourage medical advice but not control. The socially unacceptable substances (narcotics) with no performance effects should be dealt with through education and ethics. However, in the end, WADA ended up with a definition of doping where a substance or method is unacceptable if it scored on two of the three lists. This means that substances that are unhealthy and socially unacceptable are considered to be doping, even if they are not performance-enhancing. Many think WADA should have stayed with the definition of doping related only to performance enhancement and nothing else.

In relation to the problem of gene doping, it is, however, important that WADA in the autumn in 2002 introduced somatic cell doping, a form of gene doping on the list of prohibited substances. Cell doping is defined as non-therapeutic use of genes, genetic elements and/or cells which have the possibility to enhance performance in sport. WADA thereby seemed to be in front or even ahead of the development in doping. The problem is that cell doping is not possible to detect by the present detection methods.

THE ETHICAL PROBLEM IN TRADITIONAL DOPING

The ideas on which modern sport was founded when it was developed in the middle of the nineteenth century in the English upper class and at the public schools included a moral vision of how sport should function. Sports should develop the character and the personality of the athletes (McIntosh, 1979). The reasoning behind this idea seems to be based on virtue ethics. The goal was to develop virtue through sport. One would foster not only sport heroes, but moral heroes. This tradition can explain why we still seem to expect higher moral standards in sport than in other areas of society (McNamee, 1995). Elite athletes operate in a different moral category than authors, artists or circus acrobats. Novelists can use opium and philosophers amphetamine without being disgraced. But athletes are expected to be heroes and idols. Even nasal spray with ephedrine can be damaging for their status and career. However, as elite sport more and more became an entertainment industry, it became difficult to uphold the clear moral distinction between sport and the circus.

Recent elite sport ethics has therefore shifted perspective from virtue development to norm following (Loland, 2002). When fair play is seen as important in elite sport, it is because equality and justice are universal norms. Doping gives an unfair advantage that has nothing to do with what one tries to measure in competitions, namely who is best, based on talent, training and hard effort (Gardner, 1989). A narrow focus on justice and fairness can, however, lead to unwanted consequences. If it is not possible to control doping and stop the dopers, it may be better if all have the possibility to use doping if they want. That creates more equality. This means that if doping is difficult to control, the fairness argument may be used to spread doping rather than stop it (Breivik, 1992).

The norm or ethical arguments are sometimes used together with more formalistic ways of arguing based on law. There is a law or regulation against doping which the dopers do not respect. They thereby are law-breakers and cheaters. Against this one can argue that the laws are not good enough, the control apparatus is too weak. There are too few tests. And so on.

The third type of argument against doping has been arguments from a health risk perspective (Waddington, 2000). Many forms of doping can result in health damage. Against this one can argue that elite sport is not concerned primarily with health. People have a right, even in sport, to do things that are harmful to themselves. Behind this attitude is an anti-paternalistic demand for freedom to choose one's own health profile.

A more utilitarian attitude looks at doping as an extra cost. The hunt for new doping means gives advantages relative to others in the short run, but the advantage disappears if doping spreads to all (Breivik, 1991, 1992). This is a logic we know from several sectors of society. It was originally called the 'Tragedy of the Commons'. Common pastures in England were over-grazed because everybody would use as much pasture as possible for their own benefit. Some think that this hunt for advantages is part of the logic of modernity (Tangen, 1997). And it creates not only costs, but opens new possibilities.

There is also a type of argumentation that maintains that doping leads to a deviant subculture (Lüschen, 1993, 2000). Following this, one could argue that it is in the interest of sport, especially elite sport, to be part of the officially accepted culture and not become a deviant subculture. Against this one can argue that modern society and modern sport are becoming more and more pluralistic. There is a long list of different cultures, even inside elite sport.

There are some people who do not see doping as a problem. Brown (1980) maintains that the doping rules are built on a paternalistic attitude where the sport organisations try to control the athletes and their own free choices. He welcomes instead research on doping, and free dissemination of information about the positive and negative effects of doping. It is then up to the individual athlete to choose.

Brown's way of arguing displays the dilemma of the sport organisations. There are, broadly speaking, two ways to go in relation to doping. Either one must fight doping as hard as possible, with clear definitions, good and efficient control procedures and tough punishment. The other alternative is to follow Brown (1980) and let doping or not be an individual choice, but let society contribute with research, information, guidance and medical support.

GENETIC TECHNIQUES: A NEW CHALLENGE TO ELITE SPORT

Genetic manipulation is a challenge to elite sport. In international literature we often find the expression 'genetic engineering' or 'genetic enhancement' (Bouchard *et al.*, 1997). In sport the goal is to enhance performance – to improve the quality of the performer and the performance.

Genetic manipulation comes in different forms. There are three main ways of genetic manipulation. The goal may be to improve specific local functions or abilities of the performer. It is, for instance, possible to inject a gene into specific muscles or organs of the body. In the Danish doping report the authors describe three different ways of local manipulation of the body (Udvalget vedrørende doping i Danmark, 1999):

1   Direct injection of genes in the muscles. The muscle fibres will take up the gene and become modified. In this way it is possible to develop a strong tennis arm or a well-developed running foot.
2   Genes carried by virus. The virus is manipulated in such a way that the normal gene material is mixed with artificial gene material. When a person is exposed to the virus, it will transfer the artificial genes to cells in the body.
3   Injection of genetically modified cells. Cells are taken out of the body, injected with artificial genes and then put back again into the body

With the use of these techniques it is possible to affect specific muscles, but also the production of EPO or growth hormones in the body. This type of manipulation is similar to the one we know from traditional doping. Does this mean that the new techniques are nothing more, nothing less than what we find in traditional doping? Or do the new techniques raise new problems, especially ethical problems?

A more advanced form of doping will be genetic manipulation of an embryo where specific traits or abilities are modified as a result of manipulation of certain genes. Such manipulation can be carried out from acceptable motives such as prevention of certain heritable diseases. It is a small step from here to using such techniques to make athletes stronger and more robust against injuries and weaknesses. Stronger anterior cruciate ligaments, for instance, would be welcomed in many sports.

It will be far more problematic to influence specific bodily abilities to enhance performance, such as increasing strength or endurance through genetic manipulation. One could here also imagine a modification of personality characteristics or mental capacities that have specific genetic underpinnings. Toughness in ice hockey or risk taking in downhill skiing could be relevant abilities. The so-called risk gene that affects willingness to take risks was the first personality-related genet that was identified through the mapping of the human genome (Cloninger *et al.*, 1996).

Manipulation of human capacities and abilities through genetic manipulation raises complex ethical questions. Is it for instance right, as Maurice Greene asked, automatically to exclude all athletes who are genetically modified from sport competitions? Even if it happened at the embryo stage and without the athlete having anything to do with it? It is unfair to accuse the athlete. It is after all the parents, the researchers, the medical specialists, 'society' that should be accused if there is a wrong-doing. Does this mean that we then should have special classes in competitions for genetically modified athletes? How could we detect who is modified and who is not? Are there technical solutions here? Will there be in the future?

GENETIC SCREENING AND SPORT

The mapping of the human genome makes it in principle possible to identify the genetic factors that to a high degree determine performance in sport. Even if it is a difficult task, it can in the future open up possibilities of identification of sport talent already from birth or even before birth (Bouchard *et al.*, 1997). We can foresee the development of sport organisations or companies that set up programmes of screening and detection of talent, advice and promotion of sport careers. We already see tendencies for this development in some countries, even if the identification of talent is a very imprecise science at the moment. The problem with this type of intervention in the lives of newborn or small children is the question that Kant raised: Do people have a right to use other people as a means to reach certain goals? Should we not always treat people as an end in itself and does not this mean that people should themselves choose what kind of life they want to live? According to Kant and his followers, identifying talent, selecting the most promising and setting up career paths for small children is an intrusion in young people's lives that is unacceptable.

CLONING

In 1997 the Scottish cell biologist Ian Wilmut cloned a ewe, which had died six years earlier, from breast tissue cells which had been preserved in a freezer (McGee, 2000). The same year Ryuzo Yanagimachi, at the University of Hawaii, cloned a mouse, Cumulina, that produced altogether 50 copies through some stages. In November 2001 the American company, Advanced Cell Technology cloned a human cell and cultivated an embryo consisting of six cells. We are on the way to seeing a full human clone. Up till now cloned organisms have had unsatisfactory health and toughness. They are not yet candidates for being strong top level athletes. This may change in the future.

If we get human clones in the future, humans with brains, sport talent and beauty will be among the first candidates for being cloned. To freeze tissue from humans with the purpose of future cloning will become topical. Kass (2000) maintains that we soon will have commercial interests establishing 'nucleus banks' like the sperm-banks we have now. We can imagine famous athletes marketing their DNA like they now market their autographs and just about everything else. On this view, Kass suggests that cloning, if it is permitted, could soon become more than a marginal practice, simply on the basis of free reproductive choice, even without any social encouragement to upgrade the gene pool or replicate superior types.

If such a scenario is realized, we will have to decide whether cloned athletes can take part in Olympic Games or World Championships. One can imagine separate competitions for cloned athletes. One could think of eight cloned sprinters competing in 100 metre as the ultimate example of fair competition since the genetic lottery has been replaced by genetic control. We have eight sprinters with identical genetic make-up. The one who wins deserves to win because that is the person who has trained harder than the others and is more determined to win in the competition. While there still may be differences in training resources and support system, genetic inequality is replaced with genetic equality, in fact, identity. The competition will therefore be harder, more open, more exciting since it is more difficult to predict who will win. The margins will be small. One can think of this as a suitable event for both gambling and scientific research. With cloned athletes it is possible to perform controlled experiments with training, diet and psychological techniques. One could map more precisely which factors influence athletic performance. At the same time we would have to change our view about what sport competitions are about.

ETHICAL PROBLEMS

We do not know how or how fast the new genetic techniques will develop. I have suggested a few possible scenarios, but it is uncertain which direction the development will take and which possibilities will be realised. The evaluation of what to do with the new techniques will be influenced by rational arguments, by accidental facts and ethical deliberations. The actual use of genetic techniques will be dependent upon acceptance in society at large. Certain genetic techniques, for instance, manipulation of embryos, may be accepted to prevent serious diseases. Many will probably accept genetic techniques for therapeutic purposes to repair serious damage and suffering. Such therapeutic use of genetic techniques will also be accepted in sport. It is more uncertain whether a more specific sport-related use of genetic techniques to repair injuries in sport will be acceptable.

The problem will be to uphold a sharp demarcation between what is a repair of disease, injuries and defects, on one hand, and what is performance enhancement, on the other. Many therapeutic techniques will indirectly have an enhancing effect on athletic performance. A stronger anterior cruciate ligament, genetically repaired, will increase the subsequent performance of the athlete. A stronger knee makes possible tougher movements, more advanced repertoires. This may, however, be accepted. If instead it is the muscles and not the ligament that are enhanced to stabilise the knee, the case seems to be different. We now feel there is a direct improvement of performance. We are closer to traditional doping.

Some forms of genetic knowledge and genetic modifications raise, in addition, other new dilemmas. The knowledge about the human genome and the gradual identification of genes that are linked to specific behaviours will lead to a better understanding of the genetic background for athletic skills and abilities. This means that it will be easier to identify and select individuals who are well suited to specific sports. From an ethical point of view this raises the question of freedom and autonomy, of the right to choose one's life and career. Put another way, it raises the problem of paternalism where parents and coaches take the decision of how the child should live, what goals to go for, which career to choose. If individuals have the right, if persons themselves are to decide how to live, this is very problematic. Some studies show that it is better, also from a sport success perspective, if children try many sports, test themselves in many arenas, have the freedom to choose what they want with sports. Gilberg and Breivik (1999) found in a study of the most successful Norwegian athletes that they had been involved in many sports when they were kids and had gradually chosen their favourite sport and developed their career. In many ways such a model for developing top athletes is more acceptable than a model where parents and specialists choose for the child. The right to choose one's own life is fundamental.

Manipulation of embryos for athletic purposes takes the ethical questions one step further. Here humans are designed from embryonic stage with the purpose of developing world-class athletes in specific sports. The ethical focus should here be put on the people who plan and perform the manipulation, rather than on the resulting manipulated person. The general ethical problem of manipulating human embryos for specific purposes will have to be discussed in many contexts. The sports world will have to decide what to do with manipulated athletes, how they should be respected and have the chance to be involved in sport, without taking apart the idea of what sport contests is all about. Sport used to be an arena where persons by free will and out of enjoyment of sports entered the scene to test their skills against other competitors. A contest between embryonic manipulated athletes takes the contest to another level, that between the manipulators where the athletes are means and not goals.

Cloning will raise many of the same problems as manipulation of embryos. The general ethical problems will be even greater. The biological and medical dilemmas will be even harder. The recent genetic techniques and the new ways people live together have created the background for the idea of procreative liberty as a personal liberty (Robertson, 2000). The moral right to reproduce includes the right to use non-coital or assisted means of reproduction. The idea of procreative liberty may lead to the right to have various forms of cloned products of persons. There are several possibilities. Robertson (2000) suggests the following options:

(1) cloning a couple's embryos; (2) cloning one's children; (3) cloning third parties, like Olympic gold medallists; and (4) cloning oneself. There are various arguments and problems with each of these forms of cloning, but Robertson thinks that most of the problems of cloning will be solved by putting the moral and legal aspects of cloning upon the rearing of children. There should be no cloning without willingness to rear. The responsibility is then put on the shoulders of responsible persons, couples or relationships. But how responsible are these persons when there is a very talented clone and a future Olympic Gold medal in sight? One could also ask whether the right to be a full autonomous and free person is taken into account. The clone will obviously have problems with the relationship to the 'original' and the building of a separate identity as a person.

Cloning raises the basic question of what it means to be human, what it means to be an independent person. Cloning takes us to the limits of human identity and personal autonomy (Miah, 2002). A clone has not had a normal conception, has no mother and father in the normal way. On the other hand, the clone may cherish extreme skills and abilities, of being an exceptionally talented athlete with superior performance.

If one chooses a utilitarian perspective on this, the utility and skills of victories must be weighed against the costs of a weakened and staggering personal identity, autonomy and dignity. The people who planned and produced the clone, who followed it up will have costs and benefits. The people who can enjoy the superior performances of the clone will have to be weighed in mainly on the benefit side. Many people will probably also feel repugnance and disgust that contributes on the negative side, among the costs. Such utilitarian arguments and weighing costs and benefits against each other can, however, according to Miah (2002) never exceed the rights a person should have. Among such rights is maybe the right to be born and not be cloned or genetically modified. A person must have the right to make his or her own choices of steering their life in certain directions, deciding to do with their life what they wish. People should not be constructed by others for their own external purposes. This problem is emphasised with the introduction of new genetic techniques.

CONCLUSION

The article by Longman (2001) in *The New York Times* resulted in a closed meeting at the Banbury Centre outside New York where sport scientists and sport leaders met some of the leading gene researchers in the world (WADA, 2002). The researchers were relatively optimistic about the possibility of developing test methods for gene doping. This probably led WADA a short time after to put cell doping on the doping list even if at the moment no secure test methods are available. The development of traditional doping in the past ten years has led to an intensified effort, a development of new test methods, more out-of-competition testing and stronger punishment. The doping hunters seem to have caught up to the prey. At the same time there is no reason to believe that doping will stop. The hunt for advantages will lead into new areas. More advanced and refined doping methods will be developed. Doping controls will need more and more resources just to catch up. The alternative of letting doping go free, maybe under medical supervision, has few official followers among sport leaders, even if advocated by some sport philosophers (Tamburrini, 2000). Letting doping go free will, according to my view, lead to even more useless waste of resources to gain the small advantages that the others do not yet have. The pharmaceutical industry will have a golden age.

I mentioned earlier that modern elite sport is founded on basic ideas like the idea of progress, liberalism and technology. We can add capitalism. Elite sport today is a capitalist entertainment industry where the actors that have most resources, whether it is companies, organisations or countries, will win. Doping is not a one-man project, but part of the competition between systems of one type or another. This will be even truer for the new genetic techniques, if they are introduced in sport. This means that the doping problem cannot be solved by appealing to the moral sense of each single athlete. Doping can only be solved by a more encompassing project, where the larger systems and the whole sport culture are included.

In the introduction I suggested that the new genetic techniques would question what sport is all about, what competitions are for. If sport at elite level no longer involves athletes with normal biological parents but puts manipulated or cloned athletes into the arena, the whole ideological foundation of sport is questioned. If cloned athletes enter the starting blocks, the reason and purpose of competition are changed. The original idea was that normal human beings with differences in genetic make-up and differences in background, upbringing, training and social environment could meet to decide who had the best total mix and who was best on that very day, in that competition. Can we instead in the future find competitions where athletes are put into different classes and categories based on deep differences in biological and genetic make-up? The new genetic techniques give us many reasons to discuss and reflect upon the basic ideas and values in sport.

The new genetic techniques raise the even more fundamental question about what it means to be a human being. If embryos are manipulated to create sport heroes or superstars, then human autonomy and dignity will be endangered. Miah (2002) maintains that the new genetic techniques will raise questions that are so fundamental that they cannot be answered in a sport context alone. But elite sport may contribute with perspectives and insights that are important because elite sport is focused on one aspect of what it means to be human, namely, what it means to perform extremely well through bodily movements.

REFERENCES

Bouchard, C., Malina, R.M. and Pérusse, L. (1997) *Genetics of Fitness and Physical Performance*. Champaign, IL: Human Kinetics.

Breivik, G. (1991) 'Cooperation against Doping?' In J. Andre and D. N. James (eds), *Rethinking College Athletics.* Philadelphia, PA: Temple University Press, pp. 183–93.

Breivik, G. (1992) 'Doping Games: A Game Theoretical Exploration of Doping', *International Review for the Sociology of Sport*, 27: 235–55.

Breivik, G. (1998) 'Idretten som samfunnets speil', *Skrifter i Utvalg.* vol. 8. Oslo: Norges idrettshøgskole.

Brown, W.M. (1980) 'Ethics, Drugs and Sport', *Journal of the Philosophy of Sport*, 7: 15–23.

Cloninger, C.R., Adolfsson, R. and Svrakic, N.M. (1996) 'Mapping Genes for Human Personality', *Nature Genetics*, 12: 3–4.

Gardner, R. (1989) 'On Performance-Enhancing Substances and the Unfair Advantage Argument', *Journal of the Philosophy of Sport*, 16: 59–73.

Gilberg, R. & Breivik, G. (1999) 'Hvorfor ble de beste best? Barndom, oppvekst og idrettslig utvikling hos 18 av våre mestvinnende utøvere', *Skrifter i utvalg.* vol. 15. Oslo: Norges idrettshøgskole.

Guttmann, A. (1978) *From Ritual to Record: The Nature of Modern Sports.* New York: Columbia University Press.

Hoberman, J. (1992) *Mortal Engines: The Science of Performance and Dehumanization of Sport.* New York: The Free Press.

International Athletic Foundation (1997) *Human Performance in Athletics: Limits and Possibilities.* Official Proceedings, Seminar.

Kass, L. (2000) 'The Wisdom of Repugnance: Why We Should Ban the Cloning of Humans', in G. McGee (ed.), *The Human Cloning Debate.* Berkeley, CA: Berkeley Hills Books, pp. 68–106.

Kemp, P. (1991) *Det uerstattelige: En teknologi-etikk.* Oslo: Gyldendal Norsk Forlag.

Loland, S. (2002) *Fair Play in Sport: A Moral Norm System.* New York: Routledge.

Longman, J. (2001) 'Someday Soon, Athletic Edge May Be from Altered Genes: Pushing the Limits'. *New York Times.* 11 May.

Lüschen, G. (1993) 'Doping in Sport: The Social Structure of a Deviant Subculture', *Sport Science Review*, 2(1): 92–106.

Lüschen, G. (2000) 'Doping in Sport as Deviant Behaviour and its Social Control', in J. Coakley and E. Dunning (eds), *Handbook of Sports Studies.* London: Sage Publications, pp. 461–76.

McGee, G. (2000) *The Human Cloning Debate.* Berkeley, CA: Berkeley Hills Books.

McIntosh, P. (1979) *Fair Play: Ethics in Sport and Education.* London: Heinemann.

McNamee, M. (1995) 'Sporting Practices, Institutions, and Virtues: A Critique and Restatement', *Journal of the Philosophy of Sport*, 22: 61–83.

Miah, A. (2002) 'Philosophical and Ethical Questions Concerning Technology in Sport: The Case of Genetic Modification', doctoral dissertation, De Montfort University, Leicester.

Nisbet, R. (1980) History of the Idea of Progress. New York: Basic Books.

Prokop, L. (1970) 'The Struggle Against Doping and its History', *Journal of Sports Medicine and Physical Fitness*, 10: 45–48.

Ravn, J. and Hansen, L. (1994) *Sport og teknologi.* Copenhagen: Teknologinævnet, Forlaget Thorup.

Robertson, J. (2000) 'The question of cloning', in G. McGee (ed.), *The Human Cloning Debate*. Berkeley: Berkeley Hills Books, pp. 42–57.

Tamburrini, C.M. (2000) *The 'Hand of God?': Essays in the Philosophy of Sport*. Göteborg: Acta Philosophica Gothoburgensia.

Tangen, J.O. (1997) 'Samfunnets idrett', Doktoravhandling, Universitetet i Oslo.

Udvalget vedrørende doping i Danmark (1999) *Profilen: Doping i Danmark, En hvidbog*. Copenhagen: Kulturministeriet.

WADA News (2002) No. 2, p. 2.

WADA (2003) *The World Anti-Doping Code*. Version 3.0. 20 February 2003.

Waddington, I. (2000) *Sport, Health and Drugs: A Critical Sociological Perspective*. New York: E & FN Spon.

Wilson, W. & Derse, E. (eds) (2000) *Doping in Elite Sport: The Politics of Drugs in the Olympic Movement*. Champaign, IL: Human Kinetics.

Young, D. C. (1984) *The Olympic Myth of Greek Amateur Athletics*. Chicago: Ares Publishers. Incorporated.

Part V
Gender equality and gene technology in sport

15 The genetic design of a new Amazon

Claudio Tamburrini and Torbjörn Tännsjö

INTRODUCTION

Sexual discrimination is a widespread and recalcitrant phenomenon.[1] However, in Western societies, explicit sexual discrimination, when exposed, is seldom defended straightforwardly. There is one remarkable exception to this, however. Within sports, sexual discrimination is taken for granted. It is taken for granted that, in many sports contexts, it is appropriate to discriminate (distinguish) between women and men and to have men competing exclusively with men, and women competing exclusively with women. Even by radical feminists this kind of sexual discrimination has rarely been questioned. This is strange. If sexual discrimination is objectionable in most other areas of our lives, why should it be acceptable within sports? Or, does a subtle defence of sexual discrimination exist in this field, cast in gender essentialist terms?

The present authors have questioned the practise of sexual discrimination in sport.[2] We have argued that it should be abolished. Women and men should compete against one another on equal terms on sport arenas. The reasons for giving up sexual discrimination within sports, and for allowing individuals of both sexes to compete with each other is simple. In sports it is crucial that the best person wins. Then sexual differences are simply irrelevant. If a female athlete can perform better than a male athlete, this female athlete should be allowed to compete with, and beat, the male athlete. If she cannot beat a certain male athlete, so be it. If the competition was fair, she should be able to face the fact that he was more talented. It is really as simple as that. Sexual discrimination within sports does not have any better rationale than sexual discrimination in any other fields of our lives.

Our proposal has not been met with immediate and general acceptance, or even approval. Many arguments have been readily called forth in objection to our proposal. Here are some of them:

1 Sexual discrimination within sports is no different than the use of, say, different weight classes in certain sports, intended to make the result less predictable. We use sexual discrimination because we seek, to use Warren Fraleigh's term, 'the sweet tension of uncertainty of outcome'.

2   If women and men compete, and women defeat men, then this will cause violent responses from men. So we had better retain the discrimination.

3   If we give up sexual discrimination in sports, then probably all women will find, because on average they perform poorly in comparison with men, that they are always defeated by some men. This will be discouraging for women in general and for female athletes in particular.

The first argument is mistaken. When we discriminate in some sports such as wrestling between different weight-classes, this has to do with the fact that weight is a decisive factor in wrestling, that directly affects the outcome of the competition. But there exist no sports where sex is a decisive factor in that sense: sex is only indirectly related to the outcome of a sport contest. It is certainly true that there is a correlation between sex and weight, but this correlation is merely statistical. So it should not be taken into account when a system of different classes is established in a certain sport.

The second argument may be true, but it is not relevant to the question of sexual discrimination in sport. If the abolishment of the discriminatory system invites this kind of violent opposition, then this opposition should be countered by educational, punitive, and other regulatory responses. The possibility of violent resistance should not be allowed to stand in the way of a gender reform within sport, if such a reform is desirable as such.

The third argument is more difficult to set to one side, however. From the point of view of a gender essentialist feminist position, it may be tempting to argue that if sexual discrimination in sport is abolished, the immediate result will probably be that, in many sports, there are many men who can beat any woman. So we had better stick to sexual discrimination in sport. We ought to resist this argument.

First of all it should be borne in mind that to some extent the different accomplishments between women and men in sport may have to do with the fact that few women have challenged the sexual stereotypes. Thus, we have not yet seen what it is possible for women to achieve in these fields. Remember that very few women can beat the best male chess players. We do not think that this has anything to do with genetic differences. It is rather a consequence of old prejudices and a strongly established gender system. The same may be true of the performance of women in sports that require strength and endurance.

But it may also be true that, statistically speaking, no woman can compete successfully with the genetically best endowed men in these sports. If this is so, it might be thought that a system of classes based, say, on muscular mass would do the trick. However, even if this means that we need not resort to overt sexual discrimination, it may still have the effect that the classes where the best results are produced will be occupied exclusively by men.

So the best response to this argument may be to offer women the possibility of genetically becoming as strong as men. As a matter of fact, this is what we are going to argue in this chapter. We are going to discuss both whether for individual female athletes it is possible through genetic engineering to catch up with men and whether such a development, if possible, would be desirable.

Before we enter this argument it might be a good idea to consider, however, whether there exists any feasible alternative to this approach. Is there another and more conventional way of achieving gender equality within the sports? Is there something to the gender essentialist feminist position with respect to sport?

DISTRIBUTIVE JUSTICE IN SPORT

Elite sport is a male-biased activity. In the most popular and remunerative sport disciplines, physical attributes historically monopolised by males (with the exception of the mythical Amazons era) are decisive for the outcome of the competition. In the sport market, strength, muscular volume, speed and height are valued much more highly than balance, rhythm and resistance, these latter are all physical traits ascribed to a supposed female sporting condition. Accordingly, female athletes gain much less economic benefits and social recognition than their male colleagues.[3]

If we doubt that the elimination of sexual discrimination within sports will remedy this problem, at least unless we also allow women genetically to catch up with men, does any other remedy exist? The solutions usually proposed are: (1) assigning more resources to women sports; and/or (2) increasing their share of prizes and rewards above the level established by the sport market.[4]

We doubt that either of these strategies is appropriate if one really wants to promote gender equality. Proposal (1) perpetuates the division between male and female sport gender stereotypes. Proposal (2), instead, as it practically amounts to confiscating male athletes' revenues to increase those of female sport stars, would create resentment among male athletes. And even among female athletes, this move would lead to mixed feelings; certainly, those women who excel in sport want to be rewarded, but they want to be rewarded because they deserve exactly those rewards they receive; they do not want to receive out of pity or some misconstrued notion of distributive justice any more than they deserve. Therefore, instead of (1), we will promote a policy of assigning resources across gender barriers. And against (2), we will affirm the need for women to conquer powerful spaces in male, well-paid sports, not by imposed benefits redistribution, but instead, if necessary, through genetically adapting their physique to market requirements.

In her classical article 'Sex Equality in Sports', Jane English advocates equal opportunities for women in sports, without questioning what we have here called sexual 'discrimination' in sport.[5] English builds her gender essentialist feminist argument on a distinction between basic and scarce benefits of sports.

Examples of the former are health, fun, the satisfaction of doing one's best, the development of a sense of co-operation through working together with teammates, the incentive of measuring one's skills with those of opponents, improving oneself by learning to accept criticism and realising one's shortcomings.

Examples of scarce benefits of sports are fame, public recognition and economic rewards. With scarce benefits, unlike basic ones, not everyone has a right to them.

Rather, they are – or, at least, they should be – distributed according to accomplishments and proven skills. In practice, however, the allocation of rewards in professional life is strongly influenced by market appeal, which often, but not always, has a direct relation to results and proven skills.[6]

The central question in English's article is how these basic and scarce benefits should be distributed, if our goal is to secure equal opportunity for women in sports. Her answer is two-fold.

First, in the context of recreational non-professional sports and in order to secure women's formally sanctioned right to the basic benefits, sex equality in sports requires immediate changes in the way resources are distributed at present. Better coaching, better training facilities and, in general, more economic support for female sport disciplines are a necessary condition if women are to have an equal chance to enjoy the basic benefits of sports. And, if a fair allocation of resources to male and female sports is not upheld, current distribution of scarce benefits will not be fair either. How else could the best women athletes come forward and become professionals? In the absence of such concrete measures, we merely pay lip-service to the ideal of equal chances, but hardly serve it in reality.

Second, rather than depending on results and audience appeal (that is, the sport market), the scarce benefits of sports should be distributed in accordance with the idea of equal achievements for major social groups. English presents this idea as implying that a society is just if the percentage of, say, black lawyers roughly corresponds to the percentage of blacks in the population. Translated to the language of sex equality in sports, that means that 'a society is unjust if less than half its professional football players are women'.[7] However, as she believes there are apparently some permanent biological differences between the sexes in the way of that development, English proposes 'a society which invents alternative sports using women's distinctive abilities and which rewards these equally' to those of men's.[8]

Thus, taken together, English's two proposals tell us that, in comparison with men, women should not only have equal access to the basic benefits of sports, but also to professional sports activities, including the benefits of high rewards, recognition and the media coverage stemming from them, even if this requires interfering with market mechanisms.

We believe English is wrong on both accounts. English's analysis starts from the assumption that there are physiologically-grounded specific male and female sport disciplines. Today, this assumption is being questioned. Women's participation in strength-based sports increases at a remarkable pace. And as we shall see, there are means available to speed up this process. In that sense, English's first proposal is rapidly becoming obsolete. Her second proposal, the one regarding scarce benefits, is instead counterproductive. Accordingly, we will maintain that the mechanisms of the sport market should not be upset. In the next two sections, we develop both these arguments.

EQUAL DISTRIBUTION OF BASIC BENEFITS IN SPORT?

Sport is a strongly gender-stereotyped social activity. Women usually deal with sport disciplines with poor male representation, and vice versa. To a certain degree, this is obviously due to relatively fixed physiological characteristics of the sexes. But the role played in women's and men's choice of sporting activity by cultural and social factors should not be underestimated.

This gender specialisation, however, is harmful both to sports and society. It makes sport disciplines stagnate, as it constitutes an obstacle to developing new ways of playing sport games according to the characteristics of the, in relation to a particular sport discipline, the 'wrong' gender. The irruption of, say, a typically female wrestling technique is an enriching element in the socially evolving practice of sports, as well as the development of a particularly masculine way of practising synchronised swimming or gymnastics.

Also for society this 'gender division of labour' has negative consequences. Traditional stereotypes on the limits imposed on individuals by their sex are confirmed, even when there is increasing evidence that such a specialisation to a great extent rests on cultural grounds. This brings with it a lesser predisposition to try alternative professional careers, beyond the boundaries of a particular gender profile. This lack of mobility in gender barriers deprives society of valuable contributions in developing new, more efficient ways of performing social tasks.

So, even if the distribution of resources and corresponding basic benefits of sports were fair between the sexes, this does not mean that it should be gender-blind. Rather, the most rational policy, both for sports and society, is one of positive discrimination of the gender not traditionally involved in the sport discipline to which resources are allocated.[9] Shortly, in our present societies, that means more money for women who wish to practise strength-based sports, and less resources for those among them who prefer to (keep on) practising 'soft' sport disciplines. And, by the same token, the same preferential policy recommends cutting resources for males in 'big time' sports, and increasing support to male athletes engaged in female-dominated disciplines.

SCARCE BENEFITS ACCORDING TO MARKET VALUE?

Is English right in her claim that female athletes should get an equal share of rewards and recognition? We believe not, at least not as an act of redistribution. In professional sports, the value assigned to athletic performances, both male and female, is decided by the market. Whatever the reasons for this are, it is a fact that, in the best-paid sports, women do not perform at the same level as men.[10] Therefore, their performances have much less public appeal than those of male athletes. Accordingly, in order to grant female athletes similar payment, public recognition and media coverage, society would have to interfere with market mechanisms by taking a share of male athletes' revenues and giving it to women athletes. We resent this kind of redistribution.

The problem with this kind of redistribution is not that it is at variance with libertarian moral principles. According to these principles, redistributing scarce benefits would be unjust to male athletes because their products are after all the ones that generate the money in the business. But why should we accept this libertarian view?

Would rival distributive justice approaches sanction a different policy? Not necessarily. We cannot justify the kind of resource transfers English advocates by resorting to a Rawlsian approach, for instance. Even accepting that male sport stars are best off (in certain sports, promoters and managers earn more than athletes), it is obvious that female top athletes are not the worst-off group in the sports community. Rather, the difference principle supports transferring resources from elite athletes (women included) to amateur sport practitioners. Or, if we limit the range of the argument to professional sports, to those athletes who seldom win a contest or earn any money.

Nor would a Marxist perspective on distributive justice support English's argument. According to the orthodox leftist view, a distribution of resources is unjust if it stems from an unequal distribution of opportunities, mainly education and means of production. This speaks in favour of taking a share of male athletes' revenues and investing it in furthering coaching and sporting facilities for female athletes (what we might call 'the means of production' of sports). But it does not justify using those revenues to increase women's sport wages.

Yet, our reason to reject English's proposal has nothing to do with abstract principles of justice. It rests on a solid and simple pragmatic rationale. Instead of reaffirming women in the conviction that they are equally as valuable as men, we believe the kind of positive discrimination she proposes risks consolidating women's negative self-image as well as general prejudices about the possibilities of women to perform at a top level. It is one thing to level out initial conditions to yield an equitable distributive outcome. It is quite another thing to directly level out outcomes, independently of achieved results. By implementing the latter strategy, we would be risking negative reactions that the former policy does not imply. This is in our opinion a fatal shortcoming of English's proposal.

But, is it really fair to let benefit outcomes be decided by initial conditions people cannot do anything about? A somewhat different socialist approach endorses instead the injustice of a distributive scheme if it is the consequence, not only of an unequal allocation of material resources, but also of the arbitrary distribution of physiological skills and traits of personality that occurs in nature. You need not be a socialist to adopt such a view of justice. As a matter of fact, this is what John Rawls writes about this:

> Perhaps some will think that the person with greater natural endowments deserves those assets and the superior character that made their development possible. Because he is more worthy in this sense, he deserves the greater advantages that he could achieve with them. This view, however, is surely incorrect. It seems to be one of the fixed points of our considered judgments

that no one deserves his place in the distribution of native endowments, any more than one deserves one's initial starting place in society.[11]

A similar stance is taken up by one of the authors (Tännsjö) in Part II of this book. As nobody deserves what she or he is given by birth, innate traits should not be allowed to decide what share one receives of the distributive outcome. However, this is exactly what happens in professional sports. Male top athletes get a larger share of the scarce benefits on the grounds of their superior physiological traits. Or so it has been argued. But this means that we have to face the problem that, to some extent, at any rate, and statistically speaking, most women are genetically less well equipped to compete in some sports than some men. Should we allow them to do something about this?

THE GENETIC DESIGN OF A NEW AMAZON

Raising through conventional means women to the same competitive level as men in strength-based sports might be a time-consuming task, and the prospect of overcoming old gender stereotypes would remain uncertain. The same may be true of men who want to enter typically 'female' sports where balance, rhythm and resistance are decisive factors. And perhaps there are genetic barriers that cannot be overcome. So perhaps we need to interfere and allow that the process is speeded up in order to facilitate access for women to the scarce benefits of sports (and for men to have access to the even scarcer resources in typically 'female' sports). A way to move forward might be to resort to the new genetic technologies. For instance, women athletes might be offered the possibility of increasing their muscular volume through genetic modification, over and above current biological boundaries. Those female athletes who chose to manipulate their genetic structure would probably obtain an increased share of sport market revenues, comparable to the one received by their male colleagues. And, with some of them competing physically on an equal level with males, women will no longer be perceived as the 'weaker sex', either in sports or in society. Role models might therefore be expected radically to change, as a consequence of this genetically induced reduction of the difference in physical strength between the sexes. For those women who wish to do so, there will be a possibility open for them to develop a physique fully comparable with respect to strength to men's. And it goes without saying that it would also allow some men to develop typically 'female' characteristics of relevance to other sports, characteristics such as balance, rhythm and resistance. Are not these physically strong women going to be seen as 'cheats' or 'fakes'? We believe not. At worst, the first generation of Bio-Amazons might be perceived with a little bit of scepticism, but definitely not their successors. Unlike what can be expected regarding repeated interference in athletes' revenues, the public will probably get used to women's higher muscular threshold, accepting it as 'natural'.

Whatever its probable advantages, there is, however, much to be said against the proposal of genetically levelling out the muscular gap between the sexes. For one thing, it is surely felt by many that this indeed would be a risky adventure. Humans – they say – should not try to play God, changing the ways things are, and always have been, in nature. Others would instead emphasise the social risks embedded in this biological experiment, reminding us of the eugenic programme of the Nazi regime. Still others will feel prone to argue that administering medical techniques and medicines to healthy people clearly constitutes medical malpractice. Finally, other objectors, limiting themselves to a sport-based critique, argue that genetically enhancing women's physique will create more injustices in the sport arenas, as it will surely have devastating effects on fairness in competition.

All these general objections to changing the female physique through genetic engineering will be explored in the next sections. But before deciding whether this genetic programme is desirable, a more radical criticism has to be met. Some people believe that reducing the muscular gap to the point of equalising gender phenotypes is simply not possible. They see the proposal advanced in this chapter at best as an interesting thought experiment, though not technically viable, not now and not in the future either. This objection has to be met first, if we do not want our whole discussion to become merely academic.

IS THE GENETIC DESIGN OF A NEW AMAZON POSSIBLE?

A crucial point for the proposal advanced here is whether women would have more to gain from gene doping than men. Otherwise, if men could also improve their muscular volume as much as women, then the old 'natural' order would be restored and genetically modifying women's bodies would not render any benefits in the sport market. A similar question could be raised with respect to men who want to catch up with women in typically 'female' sports. Would the real women always be ahead of them?

Not to get too deeply involved in difficult empirical questions, we just assume that there are examples of sports that are, in this sense, 'typically' male and female. A conjecture we then make is that if, in a certain area, one sex is genetically disadvantaged, then, in this area, it is easier for the disadvantaged sex to catch up with the advantaged one, than it is for the more advantaged one to move further ahead. If this conjecture is borne out by realities, it means that genetic enhancement is indeed a feasible means of levelling out differences.

How plausible is this conjecture? The question of whether it is possible for women to catch up with men with respect to physical traits where men are genetically better endowed than women is of course the crucial one in the present context (even if the corresponding question about the possibility that men catch up with women in female sports is of much interest in itself). This question is difficult to answer at the present stage of scientific knowledge. Already before birth differences are established between the sexes, for instance, in skeleton and bone structure. The pelvis is different in men and women. Since the leg muscles are attached to it, the angle would be different and therefore also the maximal force possible. Some of these differences may impose limitations to what is possible to achieve through gene therapy, at least to the extent that it utilises fairly simple techniques and does not transform the body in more than a few respects. On the other hand, some other congenital differences may contribute to the possibility of levelling out physical traits that are crucial to success in sports. It might be an advantage in some sports, for example, to combine a light bone structure and strong muscles.

One consideration counting in defence of our conjecture is the following. If gene therapy were allowed, there are restrictions with respect to security on how it can be used. This means that there must certainly be limitations to what kind of changes could legally be made. A way of setting such limits would be to set limits to muscular mass, haemoglobin concentration in the blood (already implemented in some sports), and so forth. Up to a certain limit it is free for anyone to enhance his or her physical or physiological characteristics. If you go beyond this limit, you are disqualified from the competition. Such a measure would have, as a not intended but clearly foreseeable side-effect, that it would be easier for the sex that is behind to catch up with the other sex than it is for the other sex to move further ahead.

There are certainly good reasons to do with security to resort to physical and physiological limits. Once these limits are transgressed, the risk to the person who has been submitted to the enhancement increases. We know that people who have, through blood doping, training at high altitude, or EPO-doping, raised their capacity for oxygen uptake too much, risk failure of their circulatory system. It is likely that excessive muscular volume poses a similar threat to the human body. In order to avoid such risks, the upper limit should be set in a manner that does not mean unnecessary hazards to the athlete.

To resort to limitations to do in this manner with characteristics of the body of the athlete is desirable also in the sense that focus is now put on characteristics that are of immediate relevance to the achievements in the sport in question, not to characteristics that merely correlate with success.

Finally, the resort to this kind of limitation means that it is easy to ascertain whether an athlete has tried to cheat. We know that the search for prohibited substances or genetically modified genes will never be a complete success. Those who cheat will always be ahead of the controlling authorities. It is more difficult to cheat, of course, if you have to show up on the scales or give a blood sample showing your haemoglobin status. Once such limitations are in place, our conjecture gains in credibility.

IS THE GENETIC DESIGN OF A NEW AMAZON DESIRABLE?

Even if our conjecture is borne out by realities, the genetic modification of some woman to a strength comparable to the one exhibited by the strongest men might, however, be considered undesirable for a variety of reasons, some of a very general nature. One of them has to do with the risks implied in transforming the human genome. Some authors see genetic engineering as a risky business. They argue, for instance, that there is a genetic ecology, resting on a balance built into our overall genetic inheritance. If one element of that ecology is disturbed – say, by engineering the factor of strength in an individual – other genes and corresponding bodily functions might be affected negatively. Thus, according to this objection, as we do not know the results of such a biological adventure, allowing the genetic design of strong women violates a basic precautionary principle. A similar view is formulated in a Report of the Task Force commissioned by the National Council of the Churches of Christ in the United States. There they state that

> human beings have an ability to do Godlike things: to exercise creativity, to direct and redirect processes of nature. But the warnings also imply that these powers may be used rashly, that it may be better for people to remember that they are creatures and not gods.

Now, there is a religious dimension to this exhortation of caution that, although interesting in itself we do not consider fruitful to discuss in the context of this volume. And the more general arguments against genetic engineering have been discussed in many other contexts.[12] It suffices here to say that, if man was made in the image of God, and if he has been endowed with free will to design his own destiny, then that should also include the freedom to transform the human genome.

But what if transforming the human genome turned out to be much too risky? Should we not then refrain from entering into such a dangerous enterprise, independently of what religious leaders believe?

To begin with, the present objection is directed to germ-line modifications, but it does not affect somatic genetic engineering. The latter, unlike the former, will not be inherited by the off spring of the person being modified. Thus, if genetic engineering brings about negative effects, their scope will be limited to the person transformed and will not have any further effect on the human genome.

Second, the prospect of physically empowering women through genetic modification as presented here should not be understood as experimental activity transgressing previously untouched scientific ground. Rather, we think of our proposal as the inevitable consequence of the adoption of genetic technology in medicine and heath care. Thus, by the time when the making of Bio-Amazons is a concrete possibility, the techniques required will have been already properly tested. In that sense, the objection of 'playing God' has to be seen as a warning directed to the whole genetic engineering programme, not as a particular objection to its application in the area of sports. If we say 'yes' to gene therapy, then the odds are high that the reduction of the muscular gap between the sexes could be performed with the same safety – or lack of it – that will characterise standard genetic interventions in the future. Moreover, if upper limits to such things as muscular mass and haemoglobin concentration are adopted, the risks to those who resort to genetic enhancement are also limited. The objection from (unreasonable) risks therefore lacks relevance for our proposal.

THE EASTERN EUROPEAN EXPERIMENT REVISITED

Among the disadvantages that might be feared would follow from genetically programmed gender equality is the risk of recreating the Eastern European sport experiment of the 1970s and 1980s. Then East German, Soviet, and other Eastern European sports officials produced many hyper-muscled women who won numerous sport contests and were accordingly rewarded with social recognition and privileges. Some of their performances still dominate the world-best lists of the post-war era. However, although their careers were surrounded with glamour and sporting glory at the moment, we know today that their final fate was in some cases tragic. Let's not repeat this experiment in the twenty-first century! Or so could at least the present objection be formulated.

This is an impressive objection, but in our opinion somewhat misdirected. The East European experiment rested on an overt violation of athletes' autonomy, as they were deceived into believing that the medical and training programmes they were submitted to simply were standard medical procedures for elite athletes. The real nature and effects of the drugs they unknowingly were made to take were kept hidden from them.

This is, however, not the case with the genetically founded empowerment of women athletes advocated for in this chapter. This proposal presupposes full knowledge of the risks and prospects of submitting oneself to the genetic programme here advanced. Further, it rests on the inalienable right of the agent – the woman athlete – to decide for herself whether and when to undergo genetic modification. For these reasons, the comparison with the East European experiment is suspiciously biased. Rather than depending on the will of some obscure sport or political bureaucrat, the Bio-Amazons will themselves decide to transform their bodies.

Against this, some would argue that, even if in theory women athletes were free to decide whether to increase their muscular volume and physical strength genetically, this will not be the case in real-life settings. As witnessed by the current use of doping substances, there are plenty of temptations in the sport market forcing individuals to make unwise choices. The prospect of obtaining huge economic rewards, fame and social prestige, these objectors will underline, turns women athletes' decisions into non-autonomous ones.

There is a grain of truth in this argument, in the sense that all our decisions are somewhat heteronomous. Often our conduct is the direct result of social pressures and the influence upon us of different kinds of incentives. But the general validity of the present objection turns it into a trivial argument. When female athletes submit themselves to current weight-lifting training programmes to gain extra muscular strength, they are also driven by the ambition to become more successful in their disciplines. To label their conduct as heteronomous simply by the fact that they have the (socially valued) expectation of performing better at work strikes us as a rather shallow criticism. To be consistent, we should then advocate the abolishment of professionalism in sports altogether, in order to ascertain that no material incentive might be suspected to condition the conduct and decisions of athletes. And if we do that, why stop at sport? Why not abolish material incentives from our entire lives? It should be obvious by now that the present objection is wide off the mark.

THE MALE AS A NORM

There is another criticism that could be raised against our proposal, relating to what we have called a gender essentialist feminist position. According to this criticism, allowing women genetically to enhance their bodies would mean allowing women to 'turn into men'. Why on earth should they do so? According to this objection, Bio-Amazons are made, not only to adapt to male cultural values, but even to assimilate men's genotypes and corresponding physiological traits. Instead of respecting and valuing female attributes for what they are, it is proposed that women would be rewarded by their physical strength and muscular volume, in themselves male attributes. Thus, the objection concludes, males are still the ideal to strive for and females are simply expected to adapt to prevailing male norms and values. What kind of gender equality is that?, could finally be asked.

Our answer to this objection is rather speculative, but nonetheless a robust one. Who says muscles and raw strength are exclusively masculine attributes? Male physical strength is no doubt a direct result of biological factors. But are not these biological factors themselves also the result of the evolutionary history of mankind? How do we know, say, which level of testosterone males at present would have if societies had adopted more equal gender roles in the past? After all, man, like other species, is the result of an evolutionary history that could have taken a different turn, if certain circumstances had been different. It is typical of some (mammal) species that sexual differences with respect to strength are considerable (lions), while the differences are less accentuated in other species (horses). We are now at a time where we can decide about the future of the human kind. Then it is up to us whether there should be differences between the sexes in certain respects such as strength.

Who knows where the biologically given limit for female physical strength is in reality? Perhaps the muscular gap could be made much narrower, provided we change current gender patterns of conduct. And even narrower, through the adoption of the new genetic technologies.

If that surfaces now as a concrete possibility, on which grounds could males' monopoly on physical strength still be defended? In particular, if some women decide that they want to become as strong as the strongest men, why should they not be allowed to do as they see fit? This question should be addressed by anyone, irrespective of whether our conjecture is accepted or not.

Rather than sticking to gender essentialism with respect to traits that are of relevance to achievements in sport, we believe it more appropriate to conceive of gender roles and stereotypes as continually evolving. We are at present in a situation where individually, some women can decide to become successful in 'typically' male sports while, at the same time, some men can do the same with respect to typically 'female' sports. Such a crossing of barriers would be most welcome, we submit. It would do much to eliminate gender stereotypes and to liberate the individual, not only with respect to gender, but even with respect to sex.

THE ARGUMENT FROM MEDICAL MALPRACTICE

Some objectors, while perhaps agreeing with our defence of genetic engineering of women athletes, might still object that this amounts to a misuse of medical expertise and resources. Following the line of reasoning against traditional doping, opponents to our proposal will argue that medicines, and medical techniques, are to be applied to the sick; we are never justified in lending them to the healthy. As Arne Ljungqvist puts in Part I of this book:

> Virtually all doping substances are medicines, most of them obtainable only by prescription. They are intended for the prevention and/or cure of disease and/or alleviation of disease-related symptoms. Their administration to healthy young people is against basic pharmacotherapeutical principles and represents, therefore, medical malpractice.

Now, regarding medical expertise, this objection does not seem to take into account the fact that today medical knowledge and techniques are applied, not only to cure sport-related injuries, but even to enhance sport performances. In that sense, sports medicine works in a grey zone, where it becomes even more evident that the distinction between cure and enhancement is quite arbitrary. The fields of applied psychology and nutrigenomics are further examples of how knowledge from the life sciences can be, and in fact is being, applied in the world of sports.[13] Furthermore, there are examples of medicine, such as cosmetic surgery, which are today considered *lege artis*, in spite of the fact that they are not intended to cure any diseases. Also presymptomatic genetic diagnosis of diseases for which no cure whatever exists yet are being carried out at present, in many countries (for instance, Sweden) at the expense of tax payers.

If the problem has to do with medical resources instead, particularly medicines, then the present objection has to be rejected, as it implicitly assumes that genetic engineering of athletes will be financed by the State treasury. This is indeed not supported by current sports market trends. What we see nowadays is professional athletes acting as private enterprises, entering into contractual relations with different sponsors.

As a matter of fact, if we take the argument of misusing public medical resources seriously, it is not easy to grasp why tax-payers should cover the expensive and technically demanding treatment of the injuries suffered by well-paid sports stars. Let us recall that, in the vast majority of countries, present resources shortage in public health care primarily affects the poor. Therefore, there is much to argue for the proposal of making highly rewarded sports persons – both men and women – pay for sport-related medical attention themselves. And the same argument applies, of course, to genetic enhancement in sport.

Perhaps this yields even more unfair competing conditions: the rich and successful athlete will receive more effective treatment for her or his injuries. But we actually live in a sports market, where training programmes, coaching and equipment are a heavy burden on athletes' budget. Most of us, however, do not see the unfair distribution of opportunities that sponsorship gives rise to as particularly problematic. So, why should we now object to the unequal access to expensive medical treatment?

Finally, the objection from medical malpractice might be taken to mean that, whatever the arguments we could advance to convince the medical profession of the contrary, genetically engineering healthy athletes will still be perceived as a violation of doctors' code of ethics. And, for that reason, there will be many in the profession who will not wish to perform such genetic modifications. The situation might be compared to what happens in certain Catholic countries when new legislation permissive of abortive practices is enforced by the authorities.

Thus understood, then the present objection simply lacks contact with reality. As it is witnessed by the numerous doping episodes, there are at present doctors who willingly take part in the practice of enhancing sport performances, even through proscribed substances and techniques. If genetic engineering becomes widely used in medicine, as it probably will, the reluctance to resort to this kind of technology in sports medicine will no doubt be lower. We simply do not believe that, due to medical recruitment problems, a programme of genetic engineering of women athletes could not be launched.

THE ARGUMENT FROM FAIRNESS

There is a different objection to be directed against our proposal that is immanent to the realm of sports. It runs as follows: to allow the genetic modification of women reinforces unfairness in competition, as some women will become stronger (that is, more than 'naturally stronger') than their sisters. Therefore, their weaker colleagues will have no chance of winning a competition when meeting them. This is to be compared to a situation in which an athlete dopes her/himself and obtains an unfair advantage over others.

This is indeed a very common objection to any kind of performance-enhancing method in sports. The problem is that this argument already has been left behind by reality. At present, former males who have undergone a change of their sex are allowed to compete with females in practically all sport disciplines.[14] As long as we do not create a special category for transsexual athletes, the present objection to the genetic transformation of females into stronger competitors appears rather arbitrary.

One could, of course, ask why one should add one inequality to another. Perhaps transsexual athletes cannot be denied the right to compete with their newly acquired sexual identity. But this is no reason also to allow genetically modified women to compete with 'natural' female athletes: one unfair situation is enough. Or so could it be argued.

Genetically modified women do not add to the supposed unfairness provoked by the appearance of transsexual athletes in sports. Rather, they might be said to increase fairness in competition precisely because the leading sport organisations now accept former men in women sport competition. As they are physically stronger, transsexuals might be expected to be superior to 'real' women. But if we let some of these 'real' women undergo genetic transformation, at least some female athletes will now enjoy more equal competing conditions with transsexual athletes.

CONCLUSION

The upshot of our discussion should be encouraging for the programme of genetically inducing a more equal gender order in sports and society. Physically stronger women would gain for themselves a significant space in the sports market, thereby also becoming influential role models for the young. The same is true of some men who enter typically 'female' sports. And the objections that could be addressed to such a policy, we have argued, do not hit the mark. Even if it turned out to be that there will always be a difference in muscular strength between men and women, we still don't know whether this gap is big enough to prevent women from competing against men. Most probably, the muscular gap might be reduced, both by cultural and genetic action, up to the point of making sex-integrated sport competitions meaningful for both sexes. And a safe way of closing the gap that may remain would be, as we have suggested, to introduce upper limits on muscular mass, haemoglobin, and so forth, for all athletes.

Further, we have also affirmed that the risky scenario usually depicted in connection with genetic technology is exaggerated. By the time when the genetic modification of women athletes advocated for in this chapter becomes a reality, genetic technology will have been so widely tested as to become relatively safe, at least as safe as a surgical technique can get. And the association often made between genetic enhancement and racial or elitist eugenic programmes seems to completely disregard the fact that, in the Bio-Amazons' world, it is the individual athletes themselves, not State or sport officials, who decide whether or not they should undergo genetic empowerment.

If we instead turn to the objection from medical malpractice, a private, not State-financed, genetic programme can tackle this problem and even be successful in recruiting the necessary amount of medicine professionals to carry out this project.

Finally, contrary to what is feared by supporters of fairness in sport competitions, Bio-Amazons will contribute to a fairer sports world, in two senses: by allowing (at least some) women to attain rewards and benefits until now exclusively enjoyed by males, and by equalising competing conditions between them and transsexual athletes.

But, then, if the arguments advanced in this chapter apparently hold tight, why this feeling that something – difficult to point out with exactitude – is wrong with the Bio-Amazons programme, a feeling that surely many of the readers still have? Ivo van Hilvoorde provides a good answer to this in his chapter on the impact of genetic technology upon educational issues. Discussing what he calls 'a rationality of suppressing autonomy', he asserts that '[I]n a context where parents and coaches will even take the effort to modify genes, it is not hard to imagine that there would be even more coercion involved.' Something similar might be argued regarding the proposal advanced here. What kind of world are we heading for, in which women have to undergo genetic modification to get their fair share of rewards and recognition?

Well, the world that is presently being shaped will be realised independently of whether the Bio-Amazons proposal is implemented or not. In the wake of genetic therapy, enhancements in both educational skills and sporting abilities will inevitably follow.[15] The context, therefore, is already given by current progress in genetic technology. Perhaps there is something wrong with genetic technology, and this might in its turn explain the reluctance some people feel when confronted with it. If that is the case, this certainly is something that has to be shown by sound arguments. We have not come across any such arguments. And even so, the making of stronger female athletes discussed in this chapter is only a derivative circumstance in this general development. Concerning this particular aspect, we have pointed out some beneficial effects of the new technique for elite professional sports, while dismissing on solid grounds all the substantial critique of the genetic empowerment of women athletes.

NOTES

1 We use the word 'discrimination' in a neutral, purely descriptive sense. Sexual discrimination takes place whenever men and women are treated differently, no matter whether this difference in treatment is warranted or not.
2 See Torbjörn Tännsjö, 'Against Sexual Discrimination in Sports', in Claudio Tamburrini and Torbjörn Tännsjö (eds.), Values in Sport: Elitism, Nationalism, Gender Equality, and the Scientific Manufacture of Winners (London and New York: Routledge, 2000) and Claudio Tamburrini, 'The Return of the Amazons', in The 'Hand of God'? Essays in the Philosophy of Sports (Göteborg: Acta Universitatis Gothoburgensis, 2000).
3 Particularly in field and track disciplines, there might be some very successful female athletes who earn more money and get more recognition than male athletes. However, the normal situation is that, given equal level of success, males get much more of the scarce benefits of sports than females. This unequal distribution becomes even more evident in big-time sports (for instance, American Football, baseball, basketball and

soccer), where athletes are contracted, not only by sponsors, but also by a team. In these sports disciplines, there are practically no women reaching the level of reward obtained by male sports stars.

4 See, for instance, Jane English's seminal article 'Sex Equality in Sports', first published in *Philosophy and Public Affairs* 7, (3), 1978, pp. 269–77, and Betsy Postow's 'Women and Masculine Sports', first published in *The Journal of the Philosophy of Sport*, VII, 1980, pp. 51–58. Both articles are included in William J. Morgan, and Klaus V. Meier, (eds), *Philosophic Inquiry in Sport* (Champaign, IL: Human Kinetics Publishers) 2nd edn, 1995, from which quotations in this chapter are taken.

5 In Morgan, and Meier, op. cit., pp. 284–92.

6 The standard example here is the Russian tennis player, Ana Kournikova.

7 English, op. cit. p. 285.

8 Ibid., p. 288.

9 The same arguments apply, for instance, to race-blind or social class-blind allocation of sport resources. If, say, a sport discipline is widely dominated by black people, this constitutes a strong reason to support participation of other ethnic groups in the discipline.

10 At present, though it has diminished during the last decades, the average difference in men's and women's athletic records still is about 10–15 per cent. For data on this, see for instance Roy Sheppard, *The Fit Athlete* (Oxford: Oxford University Press), 1978, particularly Chapter 11: 'The Female Athlete'. Other sources on the performance differences between men and women are: Elizabeth Ferris, 'Sportswomen and Medicine', *Olympic Review*, 140, June 1979; and Eduardo Hay, 'The Stella Walsh Case', *Olympic Review*, 162, April 1981.

11 *A Theory of Justice* (Oxford and New York: Oxford University Press, 1971), pp. 103–4. See also R. Arneson, 'What's Wrong with Exploitation?', *Ethics*, 1991/2, pp. 202–27.

12 See, for example, Jonathan Glover's book, *What Sort of People Should There Be?* and John Harris's book *Superman and Wonderwoman*. Cf. also T. Tännsjö, 'Should We Change the Human Genome?', *Theoretical Medicine*, 14, 1993, pp. 231–47.

13 The field of nutrigenomics is presented in this volume by Ruth Chadwick in Chapter 10.

14 Cf. Berit Skirstad, 'Gender Verification in Competitive Sport', in Tamburrini and Tännsjö (eds) *Values in Sport*.

15 Cf. Françoise Baylis and Jason Scott Robert, 'The Inevitability of Genetic Enhancement Tehchnologies', *Bioethics*, XVIII, 2004, pp. 1–26.

REFERENCES

Arneson, R. (1991/2) 'What's Wrong with Exploitation?', *Ethics*, pp. 202–27.

Baylis, F. and Scott Robert, J. (2004) 'The Inevitability of Genetic Enhancement Technologies', *Bioethics*, XVIII: 1–26.

Belliotti, R. (1995) 'Women, Sex and Sports', in W.J. Morgan and K.V. Meier (eds), *Philosophic Inquiry in Sport*, 2nd edn (Champaign, IL: Human Kinetics Publishers).

English, J. (1978) 'Sex Equality in Sports', *Philosophy and Public Affairs* 7(3): 269–77.

Ferris, E. (1979) 'Sportswomen and Medicine', *Olympic Review*, 140, June.

Glover, J. (1984) *What Sort of People Should There Be?* (Harmondsworth: Penguin).

Harris, J. (1992) *Superman and Wonderwoman* (Oxford: Oxford University Press).

Hay, E. (1981) 'The Stella Walsh Case', *Olympic Review*, 162, April.

Peters, T. (2003) *Playing God? Genetic Determinism and Human Freedom*, 2nd edn. (London: Routledge).

Postow, B. (1980) 'Women and Masculine Sports', *The Journal of the Philosophy of Sport*, VII: 51–8.

Rawls, J. (1971) A *Theory of Justice* (Oxford: Oxford University Press).

Report of the Task Force commissioned by the National Council of the Churches of Christ in the U.S.A, 1980, *Human Life and the New Genetics*.

Sheppard, R. (1978) *The Fit Athlete* (Oxford: Oxford University Press).

Skirstad, B. (2000) 'Gender Verification in Competitive Sport', in C.M. Tamburrini and T. Tännsjö (eds) *Values in Sport* (London: E & FN Spon).

Tamburrini, C. (2000) The *'Hand of God'?: Essays in the Philosophy of Sports* (Göteborg: Acta Universitatis Gothoburgensis).

Tännsjö, T. (1993) 'Should We Change the Human Genome?', *Theoretical Medicine*, 14: 231–47.

Tännsjö, T. (2000) 'Against Sexual Discrimination in Sports', in T. Tännsjö and C.M. Tamburrini (eds) *Values in Sport*. (London: E & FN Spon).

16 Resisting the emergence of Bio-Amazons

Susan Sherwin and Meredith Schwartz

In their provocative chapter in this volume, 'The Genetic Design of a New Amazon', Claudio Tamburrini and Torbjörn Tännsjö offer a spirited and thorough defense of the provocative proposal that because equality in sports requires that men and women engage in direct competition with each other 'on equal terms in the sports arena', if it turns out to be the case that women are at a physiological disadvantage for many sports, then they should be allowed access to genetic enhancement technologies to facilitate their equal opportunity of winning such competitions. This is an intriguing suggestion, but one that we find deeply disturbing. Although Tamburrini and Tännsjö have done an excellent job in anticipating and effectively responding to most of our obections, we remain unpersuaded.

There are three major claims that we will take up. The first is the claim that '[i]n sports it is crucial that the best person wins'. The second is that gender equality requires gender sameness. The third claim we shall challenge is the assumption that such uses of genetic technology are 'the inevitable consequence of the adoption of genetic technology in medicine and heath care'.

Beginning with the claim that in sports it is crucial that the best person wins, we think it worth reflecting on the interpretation and scope of the term 'best'. In the context of sports, 'best' generally refers to the person (or team) who is best prepared and most successful at meeting the demands of the particular sport. Any competitive activity, by definition, has some measure by which success is determined and the person who most effectively satisfies this measure in a given competition will be the 'winner'. But in nearly every sporting event, the outcome is local. The person who scores the most goals, or runs fastest, or proves strongest, or displays the most grace (e.g., gymnastics), will win that particular competition. Sports are most interesting and exciting, for both participants and observers, when the competitors are fairly evenly matched such that it is difficult to predict in advance who will be the winner. Luck combines with skill, strength, training, and strategy to determine the outcome in the particular event. Sometimes, the 'best' person – i.e., the most prepared or most deserving – does not win, unless we declare that the winner is, by definition, best. Many sports events are run at local levels among competitors who are reasonably well matched and there is no sense that such activities are meaningless because world-class athletes are absent from the competition. It is simply not the case that we are always interested in identifying the most accomplished athlete anywhere in a sport. Usually, the goal is to find the most accomplished within their class. And for this, separate competitions for men and women are legitimate, as they are for different age groups (and sometimes different weight classes), and for athletes with various types of disability (e.g., the Special Olympics). We do not see why we must restrict our interest to a single winner for each particular sport when there could be two or several.

Our second concern focuses on the notion that equality requires sameness and the related assumption that, for most sports, existing male standards are an appropriate norm. Tamburrini and Tännsjö use a very wide definition of 'discrimination' claiming that discrimination 'takes place whenever men and women are treated differently, no matter whether this difference in treatment is warranted or not' (p. 196). Thus, 'discrimination' is not meant to be a value-laden term. It requires a second step to determine whether an instance of discrimination is 'warranted or not', i.e., whether or not it is morally acceptable. Yet, they then go on to say that treating men and women equally requires treating men and women the same, where 'equally' is clearly meant to be a moral ideal. In other words, they quickly collapse any distinction between same treatment and equal treatment. Yet, there is a vast feminist literature that questions whether this conception of equality is desirable.[1] Jane Flax argues, 'Indeed, the need to see everyone as the same in order to accord them dignity and respect is an expression of the problem, not a cure for it.'[2] We, too, believe that it is a mistake to interpret equality as sameness.

The principal problem with equating equality with sameness is that it fails to question the standards as they are currently set. Requiring oppressed groups to be the same as dominant groups in order to be given equal respect creates a double-bind because the group is usually oppressed on the very basis of some difference, e.g., gender, skin color, sexual orientation, or (dis)ability. Basing equality on the presumption of sameness is likely to disadvantage these people by denying the reality and implications of their difference. Since some of these differences are important to the person's identity and self-conception, and others are beyond their power to change, the suggestion that they need to assimilate to the norm that arose in their absence based on standards appropriate to the dominant group may be both impossible and offensive.

Moreover, this is not the only option available for people who desire equality. We can also restructure the norms themselves so that they reflect an appreciation of difference. Women's tennis provides an example where the unique skills and style that women bring to the game (more volleys and less reliance on an overpowering serve) are valued in their own right. Women's tennis is widely televised and often has better ratings than men's tennis. For some tennis tournaments, the women's prizes are the same as men's (e.g. the US Open and the Australian Open) while in other tournaments (most notably Wimbledon and the French Open) the wage gap remains. In tennis, there is growing appreciation of women's distinctive talents without requiring that women display exactly the same strengths as male players. This version of valuing diversity in sports has the advantage of valuing what women bring to a sport, rather than valuing only women players who demonstrate the same skills as men players. Thus, tennis offers an example of a sport that is played to different strengths and skills by men and women where both skill sets are valued and neither is 'better' than the other. We would recommend that this model be followed in many other sports.

Gender justice sometimes requires that men and women be treated differently precisely in order to ensure that they have equal opportunities. Tamburrini and Tännsjö insist that there is no reason to assume that male norms will set the standards even though, to date, most popular sports have been developed around distinctly male abilities. In contrast, we believe that the market values that determine the economic worth of sporting events are problematic since they arose within a particular social climate where male standards have long constituted the norm and the rules that are in place are generally those that suit male competitors. Without direct efforts to alter the impact of such gender bias, it seems highly likely that women will have to change to be more like men if they are to seriously compete in sports that have been designed to appeal to male tastes and strengths. Yet, Tamburrini and Tännsjö resist the idea of tampering with the existing market allocation. Their alternative is that women seek to compete in these lucrative sports 'through genetically adapting their physique to market requirements'.

This solution misses the fact the problem of oppression for women is not that men are 'naturally' superior and women are struggling to 'catch up' to the male ideal. The problem is that the construction of what is 'best' reflects male talents, and those activities that are perceived as female are systematically undervalued. We would question the assumption that strength, speed, muscle volume and height are physical traits that are superior to balance, rhythm and resistance. That they are given greater value by the market simply demonstrates that the market reflects society's sexist preference for male talents over female ones. To require women to compete on these terms seems to accept and reinforce this sexist bias. It is not leveling the playing field but protecting existing biases.

We think a better way to try to promote gender equality in sport is to try to influence (not just accept) the market, such that it no longer depends on sexist assumptions about what talents are 'superior'. That is, we want women's abilities, talents, skills, and preferences to be valued equally to those of men, whether they turn out to be the same or different. To change the market in this way would require the elimination of sexism in general, and Tamburrini and Tännsjö are right to point out that this would be a long process when compared to the 'speed' and 'ease' of genetic enhancement. We believe, however, that slow and difficult social change toward the elimination of sexism is preferable to the suggestion that women become genetically engineered to be the same as men; not the least of the reasons for this preference is that the elimination of sexism would benefit all women rather than just a few elite athletes.

Further, equality is not just about gender. The ideal of promoting equality put forward by Tamburrini and Tännsjö needs more careful attention because inequality crosses many categories of oppression such as poverty and race. Legitimizing expensive interventions for the sake of reducing gender inequality is likely to exacerbate inequality due to income both nationally and internationally. Tamburrini and Tännsjö imply that athletes would pay for these genetic enhancements themselves, rather than relying on the State treasury. They see this as a fair suggestion since lucrative sports sponsorship allows athletes the luxury of paying for elite medical services. We submit that this proposal is confounding since the genetic alterations would likely occur before the athlete had gained international success and secured these sponsorships. Indeed, if genetic engineering became the norm, athletes would require genetic enhancements before they would be able to compete at the professional level, at a time when their success is still uncertain. Surely this would create a difficulty for underprivileged children, who are already at a disadvantage in some sports that require expensive equipment and team dues. Currently, success in sports is regarded as a way out of poverty for some underprivileged children who see their poor background reflected in the history of some sports stars. If Tamburrini and Tännsjö's proposal were to become a reality, this avenue of hope may be closed, as successful athletes would increasingly come from families that could afford these expensive technologies. This problem would also be reflected internationally, where it would be unlikely that poor countries would continue to be able to enter athletes in international competition against genetic Amazons.

Our third, and most serious, concern rests with the assumption that genetic enhancement for athletic success is inevitable. First, we do not believe that such genetic alteration would be a simple matter of tinkering with a few easily identifiable genes. The more we learn about the function of specific genes, the more complicated the task of targeted, customized alterations becomes. There seems little reason to believe that genetic engineers will be able to make specific adjustments to the muscle mass of the upper body, say, without affecting hormone balance, bone density, or metabolism. In fact, given the inherent risks to such efforts, we are quite mystified as to how the human research trials required to develop accurate genetic interventions aimed at particular sports-specific alterations would ever get past research ethics boards charged with protecting subjects from unnecessary risks.

We also have difficulty seeing why this sort of biochemical body alteration would be permissible in a sports environment already struggling to hold the line against the use of chemical doping. We believe that genetic enhancement would be subject to all of the problems attached to other types of drug use in sports: there is wide agreement that it is bad for sports when competitors feel an obligation to pursue chemically enhanced alterations in order to keep up with others in their field. Without explicit restraints and a complicated monitoring and testing system, elite athletes already feel the necessity of using performance-enhancing drugs. These drugs threaten their health in both the short and the long term. For many spectators, the use of such aids also undermines enjoyment of the competition, for sports become a competition for the effectiveness of performance-enhancing substances rather than sheer human endeavor.

Why would genetic enhancement not fall victim to the same problems? Elite athletes of both genders would surely feel pressured to seek every available technology to acquire or maintain a competitive advantage despite the serious health risks likely to be attached to such practices. The standards for success would become ever more elusive for the 'ordinary' athlete unwilling to engage in such body (or mind) altering practices. Fans would feel they are watching a competition of altered humans ('Bio-Amazons') and may feel alienated from the athletes. There is, after all, little popular interest in developing athletic competitions among robots. In the meantime, the social message is conveyed to all aspiring athletes that hard work and healthy habits are not sufficient and that it is normal, even expected, to seek out medical alterations to the body you find yourself in.

In addition, we presume that to be effective, such genetic enhancements must be done at an early age – probably no later than adolescence. Can we really expect adolescents, frequently uncomfortable in their changing bodies and particularly anxious for social approval, to be in a good position to make voluntary, informed choices about adoption of genetic enhancement technologies? Already, our culture discourages most people (especially women) from believing their bodies are acceptable. Moreover, it conveys pervasive social messages that tell us we should seek out cosmetic surgery to enhance our looks, a personal trainer to improve our fitness levels, private tutors to improve our scores on academic tests, genetic testing to make sure we produce only 'perfect' children, and the means to acquire ever more money to pay for the changes needed for social acceptability. In such a climate, we are deeply suspicious of genetic enhancement being offered as one more desirable technology of personal success.

Hence, we think it is very dangerous to portray genetic enhancement as an inevitable development, treating it as already achieved and routinely accepted. Such approaches have the effect of normalizing the use of these technologies long before anyone has figured out how to make them work. It is far too early to start celebrating the coming arrival of these technologies, or even to begin resigning ourselves to their 'inevitable' appearance. Scientists and physicians are very far from being able to safely assist aspiring athletes in developing or enhancing specific genetic characteristics to give them a competitive advantage in a given sport. At this point, the dangers of pursuing such a path are significant; therefore, what is most needed is a clear statement of the reasons neither athletes nor fans should encourage their development. There is still time and opportunity to avoid their introduction if the authorities that govern elite competition take a strong stand indicating that they will not permit such interventions. It is essential that we seize this opportunity rather than celebrate creative uses of this technology.

We believe that the interesting thought experiment provided by Tamburrini and Tännsjö makes clear why sports authorities should move quickly to declare that they will classify genetic enhancement as one more form of unacceptable chemical effort at performance enhancement that will be neither recommended nor tolerated. It is possible, though by no means certain, that such a stance will have the effect that women will continue to be unable to compete successfully against men in many sports. If that is the case, we must provide the resources for women to have meaningful competition with one another and encourage fans not to treat women's sports as second rate. Like Jane English, we believe that equality requires equal resources and equal opportunity, not the requirement to change one's genetic makeup to more closely approximate the physical advantages men have for particular sports.[3] We fear that should Tamburrini and Tännsjö's proposal for equality through genetic enhancement succeed, the result will be that women will have no place left at all for serious athletic competition without risking their health (not to mention the health of any future children) and their self esteem. Such an outcome would be a step backwards, not forward, in the campaign for gender equality in sports and in life.

NOTES

1 See Martha Minnow, *Making All the Difference: Inclusion, Exclusion, and American Law* (Ithaca, NY: Cornell University Press, 1990); Gisela Bock and Susan James (eds) *Beyond Equality and Difference: Citizenship, Feminist Politics, and Female Subjectivity* (London and New York: Routledge, 1992); Christine A. Littleton, 'Reconstructing Sexual Equality', *California Law Review*, 75(4) 1987: 1279–335; and Joan W. Scott, 'Deconstructing Equality-Versus-Difference', *Feminist Studies*, 14(1) 1988: 35–50.
2 Jane Flax, 'Beyond Equality: Gender, Justice and Difference', in Gisela Bock and Susan James (eds) *Beyond Equality and Difference: Citizenship, Feminist Politics, and Female Subjectivity* (London and New York: Routledge, 1992), p. 193.
3 Jane English, 'Sex Equality in Sports', *Philosophy and Public Affairs*, 7(3) 1978: 269–277.

17 Bio-Amazons – a comment

Ruth Chadwick and Sarah Wilson

Tamburrini and Tännsjö suggest in Chapter 15 that the uneasy feeling brought about by the Bio-Amazons programme is essentially related to the issue of genetic enhancement and that this corresponds with a general unease about genetic technology *per se*. However, our response goes beyond unease to a rejection of the Bio-Amazons programme altogether. This is not because of an opposition to genetic enhancement *per se*, although there are arguments for being sceptical about technical fixes to social problems, both about their feasibility and desirability. The important thing here seems to be the context within which the argument is set: the gender issues in sport have to be considered in the light of wider considerations about fairness in this sphere of activity in particular and about social inequalities more widely. What we want to consider is where, if anywhere, does unfairness lie in relation to gender issues in sport?

First, it is important to bear in mind the extent of disagreement about the nature and purpose of sport itself, and, second, there is a particular set of issues about elite sport. The emphasis on sport as a commercial, market-led activity, or as a form of entertainment, neglects other important aspects of sport: sport may be regarded as having a social purpose (e.g. as inculcating certain virtues, such as courage and perseverance).

Too great an emphasis on the importance of winning diminishes the importance of the taking part. The concept of sport as a practice of the virtues, or as representative of human striving should not so easily be neglected. However, in so far as sport is about winning, it is a unique cultural institution, with its own rules and its own conception of fairness, what Andrew Edgar has called 'the inherent unfairness of sport' (1998: 214), whereby 'competitive sport, by its very nature, is discriminatory' (ibid.: 219). Issues about the extent to which certain groups are, in virtue of their genetic endowment, less likely to win, have to be considered in the light of this. Moreover, although sport is about winning, everyone is at some time beaten by someone else.

The thinking behind the genetic enhancement issue is that women as a group are, biologically speaking, less likely to be able to win in sports in the absence of enhancement, except in sexually segregated sport; therefore they cannot aspire to the same rewards as men can from sport. Presumably the genetic enhancement issue only becomes pertinent in the context of elite sports, but even here there are considerations which are not addressed by Tamburrini and Tännsjö which are relevant to considerations of fairness and unfairness:

1   There may be differences between different sports, but most elite sportswomen in e.g., tennis are probably capable of beating the majority of men in the world at tennis. Therefore, the problem of sex disadvantage/discrimination, if there is one, cannot be about their inability to beat men in general, nor about their exclusion, as a group, from a sphere of activity.

2   In so far as elite sports are about entertainment, arguably sexually segregated sports may attract different audiences – in other words, some audiences will prefer to watch women.

3   Even so, women cannot, apparently, in general, command the same money as men in sport. In tennis, for example, it has been argued that it is acceptable for women to earn less because women play less games: men play five sets and women only play three, an argument that is questionable on several counts: it raises the question of what the prize money is a reward for. Comparison between different sports shows that length of play, as a criterion, is not consistently applied. Test match cricket lasts considerably longer than a football match but cricketers do not typically earn as much as footballers.

Thus pay differentials are not solely based on gender. Pay differentials exist even within one (same-sex) team, e.g. in football. The 'stars' earn considerably more than others. What is the money a reward for? Entertainment value? Crowd pull factor? An incentive to encourage others to become champions? If the latter, there can surely be no argument for pay differentials based on sex differences. The basic objection for present purposes, then, seems to be that even the biggest women stars in elite sports cannot command the same attention and money as the best men. Such inequalities reflect the continuing social inequalities between men and women, particularly in terms of pay differentials in society in general, rationalised by arguments such as the 'number of sets' argument, but also arguably in terms of the valuing of those areas of activity dominated by men over those more commonly associated with women.

If this is indeed the problem then there are alternatives to the Bio-Amazons project. In principle it could be addressed through altering the reward structures; e.g., interfering with market mechanisms, but the market does not always simply reward the most talented sportsperson. It might be argued that the most watched/popular entrants to the London Marathon would have been Paula Radcliffe followed by various celebrity entrants, rather than the fastest male elite runners. A true market mechanism could, as in Nozick's (1975) example of the basketball player, operate by offering the sports star a percentage of money made from charging viewers, but this is not the system typically followed.

Another possible source of unfairness in sport is in the fact that sex is used as a criterion for stratification. Is sex segregation unfair? The view that stratification should be based on some factor which is decisive to the sport, such as weight in wrestling, ignores other ways of stratifying sports, such as the different handicapping systems that exist to allow persons of different abilities even of the same sex, to compete together, or systems that attempt to match opponents of equal ability, such as the entire football league system (or qualifying times for key international competitions). However, in the statement of Tamburrini and Tännsjö that a person's sex 'should not be taken into account when a system of different classes is established in a certain sport', they acknowledge the existence of such classification systems without following that through. While their arguments do support the case against an uncritical division of sports into men's and women's competitions, it does not therefore follow that the case for the Bio-Amazon project is proven.

In 'Fair Play in Sport: A Moral Norm System' Sigmund Loland concludes that

> There is a need to evaluate continuously what kinds of sport ought to have sex and age classes, and what kinds of sport ought not to. In these discussions, we are operating along a continuum. At one end we could have shooting, equestrian sports, archery, and sailing, in which only a degree of classification according to age among children and the elderly seems justifiable. At the other end, we could place the 100-metre sprint and power lifting, as sports where a systematic sex-and and age-classification seems necessary because of the significance of bio-motor abilities for performance.[1]

There are three possible answers, it seems to us, to the question of where, if anywhere, the unfairness lies in considering gender issues in sport:

- in the distribution of natural talent;
- in the existing reward structures;
- neither – sport is a special case where concepts of distributive justice do not apply.

As regards the first, while there are clearly differences in natural talent, this also applies within the same sex. We accept in part the view that sport is a special case, but whilst this is generally true within the context of sport itself (because it is about winning), it is not true of sport set within a social context. Segregation on the grounds of ability is arguably an essential pre-requisite to the successful playing of competitive sport: such distinctions are not arbitrary, but are part of the rules of sport itself. But inequalities in rewards or access based on arbitrary factors which reflect wider social inequalities demand justification, not rationalisation. Thus, we see the reward structures as being the area in most need of critique, and this is closely linked to questions of the social value of sport.

But after all, it's only a game . . .

NOTE

1   Part of the Ethics and Sport series edited by Mike McNamee and Jim Parry, available on www.netlibrary.com.

REFERENCES

Edgar, A. (1998) 'Sports, ethics of' in R. Chadwick (ed.) *Encyclopedia of Applied Ethics*, San Diego: Academic Press.
Nozick, R. (1975) *Anarchy, State and Utopia*. Oxford: Blackwell.

18 What is gender equality in sports?

Simona Giordano and John Harris

INTRODUCTION

Claudio Tamburrini and Torbjörn Tännsjö begin their radical and radically inegalitarian chapter in this volume with the claim that 'sexual discrimination is a widespread and recalcitrant phenomenon. However, in Western societies, explicit sexual discrimination, when exposed, is seldom defended straightforwardly' (p. 181). They suggest that the fact that there are 'women's' sports and 'male' sports is one of the ways in which sexual discrimination is 'defended straightforwardly'. They argue that, if we believe in equality, we should also believe that men and women should 'compete against one another on equal terms on sport arenas' (p. 181).

The alleged reason why women do not and cannot compete against men in most professional sports is that, due to their different body composition and skills, women would be thereby disadvantaged. In order to correct this natural inequality and to give women the opportunity to compete with men on equal terms, we should enable women to 'genetically adapt[ing] their physique to market requirements' (p. 183). Women then should be given the chance to modify their genome to become as physically gifted as men, and then allowed to participate in competitions with them.

It is very important to stress here that Tamburrini and Tännsjö are concerned with gender equality, non-discrimination and distributive justice. It is important to stress this because, as we are now going to show, their arguments are in fact discriminatory, and reveal a male chauvinist ideology. We shall also discuss the way Tamburrini and Tännsjö equate equality with the idea of 'ability to compete on equal terms'. In the final part of the paper we shall briefly discuss the fact that sportswomen are often economically disadvantaged compared to men in sports. Moreover, we shall argue that the attraction of sports relates to a number of different skills, and that the beauty or artistry of many sports relies on what the individual can achieve by his or her own authentic means. Finally, we will suggest that promotion of equality in sports should be understood in a different way from that proposed by what Tamburrini and Tännsjö. Our concern for equality should not be addressed to correcting physical inequalities: a better way to be preoccupied with equality is to promote sports and physical activities in larger strata of population, to discuss ways in which everybody – regardless of sex, age, ethnic or social background – could be enabled to participate in sports, exercise and physical activities.

EQUALITY IS COMPATIBLE WITH BOTH LEVELLING UP AND LEVELLING DOWN

Tamburrini and Tännsjö wish to appear as the 'knights errant of gender equality in sports'. They represent themselves as the defenders of gender equality and non-discrimination against women. Their arguments might well look attractive to the superficial reader concerned with women's rights since Tamburrini and Tännsjö hold themselves up as champions of the 'gender battle' in the sports arena. They are fighting for a better world where men and women are treated more 'equally'. However, their conception of chivalry is an odd one, for them the mission of a knight errant is to rescue ladies who are not in distress and eradicate them! A strange chivalric mission indeed!

They begin their piece by complaining about a number of 'injustices'. Women are excluded from male games (sexual discrimination); even in the same sports, women get paid less (distributive injustice); often they get less fame (sexism).

Tamburrini and Tännsjö denounce this as one of the ways in which sexual discrimination is 'defended straightforwardly' and in addition suggest a solution to this ethical problem. The solution would be to offer women the possibility to genetically 'enhance' their body, and to enable them to physically compete with men. The physical enhancement would allow them to compete 'on equal terms'.

Despite their presumably good intentions, both the way they present the problem and the solution suggested in fact reveal a tendentious attitude towards women. Tamburrini and Tännsjö argue that in order to promote equality in sports males and females should be allowed to play against each other. Genetic engineering would offer the possibility to correct the natural inequality between men and women. It would allow women to get a 'stronger' physique, adequate to the competition with males. Science should be employed to correct natural 'deficits', an example of how nurture improves nature!

Now, if equality and non-discrimination were the real concern here, the argument might take another direction. Tamburrini and Tännsjö could have argued, for example, that in order to correct the 'natural' inequalities between men and women, males should be required to have much less training than women, or no training at all. Or that men and women's training should be monitored in order for them to get very similar strength, endurance, and so on . . . or if science should be employed, Tamburrini and Tännsjö could have argued that men should be given drugs to make them weaker or less skilled or that their genome should be modified in order for them to become more similar to women in the way that is relevant to restore equality.

Equality, in other words, is compatible with both levelling down and levelling up. In order to abolish the distinction between male and female sports, we could make males weaker, rather than women stronger. Why do Tamburrini and Tännsjö not argue for this?

Of course there is something immediately tendentious about using terms like levelling down and levelling up in this context. Perhaps one should more cautiously simply say that where inequality exists there is always more than one way of levelling the playing field if that is what equality appears to demand. However it is our contention that in this context equality requires no such thing.

HOW TAMBURRINI AND TÄNNSJÖ'S ARGUMENTS HIDE A MALE CHAUVINIST IDEOLOGY

Tamburrini and Tännsjö presuppose, without argument, that it is a certain set of typically male qualities that equate to excellence in sports. This is by no means necessarily true, and would require arguments which Tamburrini and Tännsjö do not produce to make the claim even plausible.

However, the main problem with Tamburrini and Tännsjö's piece is that, behind an appearance of equality and non-discrimination, a male chauvinist ideology is hidden. The reason why Tamburrini and Tännsjö do not argue for 'levelling down' is that they are not concerned with gender equality or non-discrimination. Or, maybe they are, but in the battle for equality, it is women who have to equate to men.

We may make our point clearer with an example. Disabled people may participate in sports and competitions, but normally they have their own games. The relationship between the classic Olympics and the 'Para-Olympics' is in a way similar to the relationship between men's and women's sports. Not that being a woman should be regarded as a 'disability'. The parallel is that, because of their physical differences – or different abilities – these two groups have separate competitions. If we were (or had to be) primarily concerned with equality, and if equality had to be served by making people 'physically equal', then we would have a moral obligation to disable 'normal people'. If equality were or had to be our primary concern, in fact, we had to recognise a moral obligation to level the physical inequalities and to allow everybody to compete against each other on similar grounds. Given that we cannot at present cure many disabilities (such as spinal cord injuries), we would have a moral obligation to disable those who can walk, so that the difference in physical abilities would be corrected and equality would be restored in sports arena. This is a conclusion that most people would surely find repugnant.

The fact that we do not regard ourselves as having a moral obligation to disable everyone seems to show that we are not primarily concerned with equality (at least, with equality meant as equality in physical capacities – a point that Tamburrini and Tännsjö fail to recognise is that equality among people might not be served by making them physically equal. We will discuss this in the following section). Indeed, we prefer to maintain inequality. We believe that most of us – at least those who are not disabled – would not commit themselves to a principle of equality that requires that they be made paraplegic.

Elsewhere one of the present authors has characterised disability as follows.[1] A disability must first be in some sense a harmed condition, and, in addition it must also be a condition which a reasonable person would have a strong rational preference to avoid. While disability normally understood qualifies on both these counts, gender does not. To be a woman, as women are presently constituted, is neither to be in a harmed condition nor is it to be in a condition that a reasonable person would have a strong rational preference to avoid. But, however disability is defined, whether for example as a departure from 'normal species functioning' or from 'species typical functioning', following Boorse and Daniels, for example, being a woman would not qualify as in any sense disabled.[2]

The ideology behind Tamburrini and Tännsjö's suggestion presupposes distinctively male attributes as the equivalent of 'health' and 'wholeness' in body. Many disabled groups reject the idea that the non-disabled embody a better paradigm of the good life. But even if we disagree about this, there are few today who would judge that the embodiment of masculinity is better *per se* than the embodiment of femininity. The fact that they suggest that women should be allowed (or encouraged?) to make genetic modifications to their body (rather than the other way round) shows that they are implicitly endorsing a male chauvinist and sexist ideology.[3]

It is not by chance that they use terms like: 'it is possible through genetic engineering to catch up with men' (p. 188). Not that there is something immoral a priori in using biotechnology to modify our body. We agree with Tamburrini and Tännsjö that objections such as those that might be encapsulated in the slogan: 'this would mean playing God' do not justify interference with private choices (choices made by individuals and affecting them only). We are contesting the idea that Tamburrini and Tännsjö's suggestion is made for the sake of equality. Tamburrini and Tännsjö's ideology is, on the contrary, profoundly inegalitarian. It is one in which the 'preferable' attributes are the masculine ones, the ones to aim for, the ones for which it is worth undergoing medical procedures in the form of genetic modification, an ideology in which equality should be restored and women liberated by 'enhancing' the female physique.

THE IDEA OF 'COMPETING ON EQUAL TERMS'

The second point we would like to address concerns the meaning of 'equality'. 'Equality is a popular but mysterious political ideal'.[4] In spite of the many philosophical inquiries into the meaning of equality, and into what it means to treat people according to the principle of equality, it is clear that the moral force of appeals to equality derives not from notions of equal competition or equal opportunity, but rather from the obligation to treat people with equal concern and respect.[5] Thus the appeal to equality necessary to sustain the particular interpretation given to equality by Tamburrini and Tännsjö would require an elaborate defence of a distinctive conception of equality. Whilst we recognise that such a defence is both beyond the purview of Tamburrini and Tännsjö's chapter and our own, it is probably sufficient to point out that the idea Tamburrini and Tännsjö employ of competing on equal terms is the least promising conception of equality to employ in this context.

The problem with Tamburrini and Tännsjö's argument is that they claim that in order for us to respect people's equality, we should make them 'equal' by eradicating their physical inequalities. This conception of equality has been forcefully and convincingly contested a long time ago by Rousseau.

Nearly 30 years before the French Revolution Rousseau offered one of the most important declarations of 'equality' of all times (1789). Jean Jacques Rousseau pointed out that the notion of equality may have different meanings, and that it is important to clarify what we mean by 'equality'. For example, saying that 'men are equal' does not of course mean that they are 'physically' equal ('in strength or intelligence'), but that they are 'morally' equal (in rights and by convention).[6] In his *Du Contract Social*, we read:

> Je terminerai ce chapitre et ce livre par une remarque qui doit servir de base à tout le système social; c'est qu'au lieu de détruire l'égalité naturelle, le pacte fondamental substitue au contraire une égalité morale et légitime à ce que la nature avait pu mettre d'inégalité physique entre les hommes, et que, pouvant être inégaux en force ou en génie, ils deviennent tous égaux par convention et de droit.
>
> (Book 1, Chapter IX)[7]

I shall end this chapter and this book with a remark that will have to be used as the ground of any social system: that is, that, instead of destroying natural inequality, the fundamental covenant will substitute, on the contrary, a moral and legitimate equality, to the physical inequality that nature may have set up among men, and that men, who may be unequal in strength or intelligence, become equal by convention and legal right.[8]

It is clear that in order to treat people according to equality we should not strive to make them physically equal, as Tamburrini and Tännsjö suggest. Rather, we need to celebrate the differences that obtain between human beings and ensure that, despite these differences, individuals are not disadvantaged. We simply should not attempt to eradicate those 'inequalities' that are not intrinsically harmful and that many of us regard as making life more rather than less worthwhile.

In contemporary philosophy, Ronald Dworkin provided further clarification of what it means to treat people according to the principle of equality. Dworkin argued that to respect people's equality is to show them equal concern and respect, rather than simply to treat them the same.[9] Putting people in the position to compete on equal terms while making them in a sense equal may well be to deny them equal concern and respect, precisely because, far from according respect to them for whom they are and for what identifies them as persons, they would be respected only insofar as they have the physical attributes that enable them to compete with others similarly endowed.

DISTRIBUTIVE JUSTICE

Tamburrini and Tännsjö complain that:

> Elite sport is a male-biased activity. In the most popular and remunerative sport disciplines, physical attributes historically monopolised by males . . . are decisive for the outcome of the competition. In the sport market, strength, muscular volume, speed and height are valued much more highly than balance, rhythm and resistance, these latter all physical traits ascribed to a supposed female sporting condition. Accordingly, female athletes get much less economic benefits and social recognition than their male colleagues.
>
> (p. 183)

In their chapter, this is presented as 'an ethical problem': one of discrimination against one sex. It seems to us that this is, however, not an ethical problem, at least not an ethical problem of injustice. The fact that male activities are paid more depends on the public's preference for those activities. There is nothing unjust in the fact that the public prefers male football to female football. There is nothing unjust in the fact that, because the audience is larger, sponsors are willing to fund male football rather than female football. The audience is larger, the 'market demand' is greater, and consequently the financial benefit is proportionally higher. This is an aspect of a capitalistic society, where prices and financial benefits depend (to a large extent) on the balance between demand and supply. Chess players get paid less (if they get paid at all) than footballers, because, so it seems, very few people would turn on their TV to watch a chess tournament. The same goes for 'push-pin'[10] and for many other classes of competitors and competitions. Musicians in the world's major orchestras probably get paid less than David Beckham. All these do not seem to be ethical issues – at least not issues of justice. These are facets of capitalism and liberal economy, in which prices are determined (to a large extent) by economic forces, one of which is the audience or the preferences of the majority. An objection to this particular inequality in 'wages' would thus entail a critique of the capitalistic economy altogether. Not that capitalism is unobjectionable. However, the implications and the scope of their critique of distributive injustice are something that Tamburrini and Tännsjö have not considered in their paper.

THE BEAUTY OF SPORTS

The assumption behind Tamburrini and Tännsjö's argument is that the essence of all sports in which male physiology gives an advantage over female physiology is located in that difference in physiology, correlating with a combination of strength, speed and muscular volume. It is not clear to us that the spirit of football or cricket or rugby or swimming consists in the role played by strength, speed and muscular volume. On the contrary it consists of many other things, including technical skills, grace, artistry, style and many other qualities. It is true that grace, artistry and style are sometimes and in some sports or activities paid less, but this does not seem to us a good reason to eliminate them from earth – or even to encourage their elimination. This is to surrender to the market logic and to convey the idea that female specific traits – because they are paid less – are not worth being pursued and had better be manipulated.

Moreover, it seems to us – although we realise that this is perhaps rather a personal opinion, than a philosophical argument – that the beauty and artistry of sports are related to the individuals' capacity to achieve the best that they can given a particular physical constitution and the particular level of skills and ability that can be accomplished through hard work and dedication. A robot running 100 miles per hour would not elicit any admiration (we would instead admire the inventor, for what he or she has been able to create). What we admire in sports, it seems to us, is what people can achieve by working on their body by their own means. This is also why anabolic steroids or other drugs enhancing performance are generally regarded as 'cheating'. Tamburrini and Tännsjö's suggestion would thus, in our opinion, undermine the very essence of both the beauty and the point of sports.

WHAT IT IS TO BE CONCERNED WITH EQUALITY AND NON-DISCRIMINATION

We believe that a better way of being concerned with equality and non-discrimination is to direct our efforts to deliver sports and physical activities to more people and to a wider strata of the population. Tamburrini and Tännsjö touch this point when they discuss Rawls's Difference Principle. According to this principle, a rational agent would choose to live in a society in which resources are spent to ameliorate the condition of the least well off.

It seems to us that sportswomen are not the least well off in our society. The main problem of inequality and discrimination in sports, exercise and physical activity concerns the fact that physical activity and sports are still a sort of luxury that many people cannot afford in terms of money and time.

Often people with low socio-economic status, or aged people, do not have the capacity to access sports or even physical activities of various sorts. This is due to lack of facilities, lack of information about the importance of exercise, lack of time and money. This is an inequality and a form of discrimination, the eradication of which, we believe, should have the highest priority.

The scarce opportunities that many people, especially older people and people with low socio-economic status have to access sports and exercise activities has a significant impact on public health. The major causes of death in industrialised countries (heart diseases, cancer, diabetes) are preventable conditions, and an essential part of prevention is physical activity. Recently the connection between obesity and these and other causes of ill health has been highlighted, and this too is connected to physical activity and indeed to sports.[11]

Serious concern for equality and non-discrimination in sport should lead us to discuss means to encourage and deliver physical activities and sports in a way that is affordable and available to everybody.

CONCLUSION

The issue of equality and non-discrimination in sports and exercise is indeed an important problem that needs to be addressed. However, we believe that the problem does not lie in the fact that women and men have different games and competitions. Tamburrini and Tännsjö's proposal is misleading, in that it appears as being in reality inegalitarian and discriminatory against women.

We believe that gender differences should not be corrected, and that females and males appropriately participate in competitions with competitors who are similarly skilled. It seems to us that the fact that there are male and female sports and exercise activities is in no way discriminatory or an offence to equality. People can still and should still be treated with equal concern and respect regardless of the tournaments in which they participate, regardless of their physical differences or genetic structure. Gender, and what it entails in terms of physical capacities, is not an element that requires medical or genetic remedy. In so far as gender constitutes 'a disadvantage' in some contexts this is purely a contingent matter. It is, in short, a social, political, economic and moral problem requiring social, political, economic and moral solutions. To offer a medical or a genetic solution exacerbates the problem and insults women. It would be the equivalent of proposing a remedy for racism which involved a genetic alteration in skin pigmentation rather than a comprehensive assault on prejudice and unfair discrimination.

NOTES

1 See John Harris, *Wonderwoman and Superman* (Oxford: Oxford University Press, 1992) and his 'One Principle and Three Fallacies of Disability Studies', *Journal of Medical Ethics*, 27(6), 2001: 383–8.
2 Christopher Boorse, 'On the Distinction between Disease and Illness', *Philosophy and Public Affairs*, 1975.
3 A similar point is also made by Sherwin and Schwartz in their commentary, 'Resisting the Emergence of Bio-Amazons' (Chapter 16 in this volume). We think, however, they have missed the central point, which is the fact that the suggestion itself reveals a strong ideology in favour of 'being a male'.
4 R. Dworkin, 'What is Equality? Part 1, Equality of Welfare', *Philosophy and Public Affairs*, 10, 1981: 185–246.
5 See R. Dworkin, *Taking Rights Seriously* (London: Duckworth, 1977).
6 Simona Giordano, 'Health Care Rationing: Demographic Revolution and Inescapable Consequences?', accepted for publication *Cambridge Quarterly of Health Care Ethics*.
7 J.J. Rousseau, *Du Contract social, ou Principes du droit politique.* (Amsterdam: Chez Rey MM, 1972).
8 Translated by Simona Giordano.
9 Dworkin, op. cit., pp. 227ff.

10 'Prejudice apart, the game of push-pin is of equal value with the arts and sciences of music and poetry. If the game of push-pin furnish more pleasure, it is more valuable than either. Everybody can play at push-pin: poetry and music are relished only by a few', Jeremy Bentham, *The Rationale of Reward*, Book III, *Reward Applied to Art and Science*, Chapter I, Art and Science – Divisions (R. Heward, London, 1830).

11 See Simona Giordano, 'The Ethics of Health Care Distribution in Europe', website available at http://les.man.ac.uk/simona/. See, in particular, 'Physical Activity and Ageing'.

Index

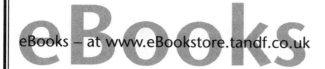